"At last a seasoned and highly trained front-line physician has written a book that provides the theory and framework to successfully integrate arts therapies and arts environments into the contemporary hospital setting. This book is a creative combination of solid research, poignant and instructive patient narratives, and practical tools that can be implemented immediately. Written by a doctor with great skill in a branch of medicine that demands the best that modern science and compassion can offer, this book will drive a much needed, broader acceptance of responsible, professional, and effective hosptial-based Arts in Medicine programs."

—Dr. Rick Lippin

"This book is a work of art on a foundation of important, valid, and sound scientific information. It is the finest expression of how to practice holistic medicine, by integrating the body, mind, and spirit, and promoting health through wholeness and creativity. I believe that by reading this book, both patients and practitioners will bring about improved health and creativity, and a higher quality of holistic health care."

—Lance S. Wright, M.D., Professor of Integrative Medicine and Psychiatry at Capitol University of Integrative Medicine in Washington, D.C., and Founding Member of the American Holistic Medical Association

Illness and the Art of
Creative
Self-
Expression

Stories and exercises from the arts for those with chronic illness

JOHN GRAHAM-POLE, M.D.
FOREWORD BY PATCH ADAMS, M.D.

New Harbinger Publications, Inc.

Publisher's Note

This publication is designed to provide accurate and authoritative information in regard to the subject matter covered. It is sold with the understanding that the publisher is not engaged in rendering psychological, financial, legal, or other professional services. If expert assistance or counseling is needed, the services of a competent professional should be sought.

Distributed in the U.S.A. by Publishers Group West; in Canada by Raincoast Books; in Great Britain by Airlift Book Company, Ltd.; in South Africa by Real Books, Ltd.; in Australia by Boobook; and in New Zealand by Tandem Press.

Copyright © 2000 by John Graham-Pole
New Harbinger Publications, Inc.
5674 Shattuck Avenue
Oakland, CA 94609

Cover design by Blue Design
Cover photograph by Allen Cheuvront
Edited by Heather Garnos
Text design by Tracy Marie Powell

Exercise on page 25 adapted from *Thriving* by Robert S. Ivker and Edward Zorensky, © 1997 by the authors. Reprinted by permission of Crown Publishers, a division of Random House, Inc.

Exercise on page 84 adapted from *A Creative Companion,* © 1991 by SARK. Reprinted by permission of Celestial Arts, PO Box 7123, Berkeley, CA 94707.

Library of Congress Catalog Card Number: 99-75297
ISBN 1-57224-202-7 Paperback

New Harbinger Publications' Web site address: www.newharbinger.com

02   01   00

10   9   8   7   6   5   4   3   2   1

First printing

For Sheila, Geri, George, and Kate

Contents

Foreword

Art is an essential nutrient for human culture. Every society has used art to create a social glue, to express its faith and ideas, and to interpret the world. There have been members of communities who have made artistic expression their life's work, while the rest of us put creative expression into our day-to-day lives for our own pleasure.

Our current economic system has disconnected art from the general public. Art now is seen as something either with a huge price tag or as a failure, without connecting it to the simple joy of creation. One hears on all sides: "I'm not an artist." In schools, art programs are the first to be cut for budget considerations. The reasons for the diminishing focus on art are several: There are few ways to judge the quality of its expression, and very, very few can make a living at it. This century of electronic wizardry, with its radio, TV, and computers, has dramatically diminished the amount of time people give to artistic expression. Manipulated consumerism has laid another blow on creativity by encouraging people to go and buy many things they used to make for themselves.

The consequence of this social disconnection from the arts is the malaise we physicians see as so pervasive in our society. I find a frightening lack of self-esteem in our adult world. People are so unsure of themselves that you hear of workshops you can go to to find your authentic self. The amount of boredom, loneliness, and fear in our society is so massive that it seems to have become our steady state. The quantity of psychopharmaceuticals being prescribed only serves to back this up.

I started out by saying that creative expression, or art, is an essential ingredient of human culture. In fact it is an essential part of being human. So how can we return art to our everyday life? How can we introduce art-making to people safely and have them listen? John Graham-Pole shows us precisely how in this book. Here are the ABCs of personal reconnection to artistic expression—accompanied by that great seducer: "It's good for your health." John tells each and every one of us: "You are an artist, and making art in any and all its forms will be good for you." He shows—without academic and scientific baggage—that personal artistic expression can bring meaning to your experience of illness as well as be potent preventive medicine. I feel like I'm in the presence of a grade-school teacher introducing to his lads and lasses the enchantment of creativity—not only its product but also the absorption and magic of its creation. Get out your crayons, your kazoo, and your dancing shoes and *go do*.

All we are saying is: Give art a chance. John's years around profound childhood illness and his love of the arts filter through his tender childlike nature to express themselves in this book. You just want to get down on the floor and *make something*. Judgment be damned: Dare to take the plunge, cast off your accustomed roles, be vulnerable, and see the world and yourself with fresh eyes.

This century has pushed compassion, humility, mystery, and joy out of our health care system in favor of corporate medical *business*, where the bottom line is profit, not care. For thirty years now, the arts have tried to bring these back into the health care system—but through the back door. Deep down, everyone knows the value to their health of music, art, poetry, clowning, and dance. But our society just hasn't made the crucial link and decided to put these treasures into every health care setting on their own merit. Each art form has been separately developed as a "therapy" practiced by a very few specialists, with narrowly defined guidelines, because this is the language the administrators of health care speak and understand. I find it enormously limiting to regard creative self-expression as a prescribed therapy that a few specialists can bill for. I hope that those who consider using art in any of its many magical forms in their healing work will open themselves to the infinite number of ways in which it can be done. Invite artists to pass through the front doors of every health care facility to do their work of healing.

Because creativity is great medicine for all, both the creator and the one who experiences it. It prevents disease and promotes wellness. It is not an indulgence, it is fundamental to medical practice. There is no universe more boundless than that of the imagination. It gives us our wonder at the world around us, our curiosity and improvisational skills, our sense of play, and our sharing of ideas. The artist is peer to the doctor. Art uplifts, educates, brings beauty, and facilitates social change. Bringing imagination to our every endeavor makes us happier and healthier. But imagination becomes flabby if not exercised. I urge you not to neglect it.

Thank you, John, for creating this book. I will hand it to both caregiver and care recipient and tell them: "Feel the wealth of possibilities for exploration. Try every exercise many times. Do them with friends. Make them fun. Turn off your TV and spend the day as a creator. You'll like where it takes you, so make creating a part of your life." This is not just a primer—it's a kick in the pants.

—Patch Adams, M.D.

Acknowledgments

My grateful thanks to my friends and colleagues at New Harbinger Publications; to Maureen Preuss, my secretary and teacher extraordinary; and to Patch Adams, dear friend and fearless evolutionary probe.

Introduction

Why I Wrote This Book

I've been hanging out with children most of my life, man and boy. In fact, I've spent thirty-odd years caring for children with cancer and their families. Some people think this must be soul-destroying work, but it's not at all. These tens of thousands of young people have been my inspiration. They've given me much more than I could ever give back. They've shown me time and again how you can face up to a life-limiting illness with courage and creativity. They inspire each other and everyone around them. Often they seem to carry their own families through.

How do they do this? By living in the moment. Children don't lurch—the way we adults so often do—from past regret to future anxiety, totally missing the bit in the middle: our precious gift of the present. They are *artists* in life, relishing each minute for the juice they can wring out of it. As artists they know to turn often to the rich resource of art-making—painting or song, poetry or dance—whenever they need to make sense of scary or confusing things, whenever they want to relax and have fun, and especially whenever they need help finding words for things they have a hard time expressing.

If children can do all this so easily, I asked myself, why can't grown-ups in similar circumstances? So ten years ago, inspired by my child-patients' example, I started a program at my hospital called Arts in Medicine. I wanted to capture these young ones' zest and creativity, bottle it like medicine, and dose it out to adult patients, so many of whom seemed to have lost this creative inspiration.

But I couldn't ask the children to get out of bed and become the grown-ups' teachers. So instead I and my friend and colleague, nurse-painter Mary Rockwood Lane, called on artists from our community and university. We knew their continuing involvement with art had kept them in touch with the artist-child within them. We hoped they could bring this healing medicine to the bedsides and clinics of grown-up patients, and show them what it could do for their *total* health—that of their body, mind, and spirit—no matter what was ailing them.

The result is this practical book that distills what I've learned. In these pages you'll find out how you—an adult, perhaps with a serious illness or disability, or maybe caring for such a person—can put art of all kinds to work for you, for your greater health and well-being.

Bringing Art Back into Your Life

You'll discover easy ways in which you as a "nonartist" can make art once more. A regular "dose" of art-making can, I firmly believe, make you healthier and happier. This is especially true if you are dealing with serious illness, disability, or any long-term adversity. I mean by *nonartist* anyone—it's actually the great majority of people—who doesn't have special training or expertise in a particular art form: painting or poetry, music or dance. The truth is, though, we're all natural artists—always have been, always will be. What this book offers is not so much works of art as *art that works*.

Every one of us as young children was urged by our parents, as well as our kindergarten and early grade teachers, to make art of all kinds. And you took to it with relish—without any hang-ups or worries about whether you could do it *right*. You went at it for the pure fun of giving voice and expression to your true and natural self in endless different ways. No one was looking over your young shoulders, judging the quality of your work. But all too soon came the day when it was time for you—unless you were one of a tiny percentage of people—to put these trivial things behind you. It was time to get on with the *serious* business of learning, and of *getting ahead* (which you might also think of as *getting a head)*, letting your thinking and judging left brain take charge. Art just wasn't an option for you if you were to make a living.

The Critic

If you do happen to be one of those rare ones who persisted into adult life with practicing some art form or other, getting professional training and so on, then for sure you too had to take life very *seriously*. The pure fun of art-making you delighted in as a young child most likely got lost early on in another version of *getting ahead* and beating the opposition, just to satisfy your everlasting critics. Just like the nonartists, your career became an endless slog of studying and concentrating and practicing, just to keep your head above water.

Julia Cameron, in her book *The Artist's Way* (1992), refers to the Censor that we all have squatting there inside our calculating and judging left brains. This is your internalized perfectionist, the carping critic that finds fault with your every effort at creativity. It may have the voice of your parents or your first-grade teachers, your older siblings or your schoolmates. It may roll all of these into one. It's very rare to be free of this inner critic, no matter how good you get at anything. But the crucial point is that it is *internalized*—that is, it was put into you from outside. It wasn't there to start with.

So I suggest that if an illness or disability has come along to slow you down, spinning your life out of your own control, but also perhaps leaving you with a little time on your hands, then this is the *perfect* time for you to reclaim that very young child within you all over again—before the censor ever entered in there. Wouldn't you like to be once more that natural artist-child who was praised and encouraged, that no one ever judged or criticized? Because that child-artist really is waiting patiently within you, in your artistic right brain that feels and intuits and imagines. Your artist-self is eager to leap out and show herself once more, in all her many shapes and shades and patterns.

If you do invite her back into your life again, I promise it will serve you well. She will help you shape and express your every emotion, especially those half-formed and confusing notions you find hard to put into words. She'll let you take back once more the delight that comes from focusing on this present moment. She'll recapture for you the endless joy of dabbling and doodling, of playing and inventing, of putting your endless imagination to work. These are the things every child does instinctively. And I'm going to make it my business to help you overcome any reluctance you may have to indulging yourself in this way. I'm going to give you permission to joyfully make art once more.

New Ways and Old

All of us have had acquaintance with hospitals, and with other places where health care is delivered. This book is especially slanted toward those of you with health problems and your families. You the reader may well be in a hospital right now, or else be a regular attendee at one. Today's hospitals are twenty-four–hour places, like police stations and prisons, fire and rescue services, all-night cafes and grocery stores. Actually they've got a bit of all of these: their own police and phone switchboard, mainframe computer and helicopter pad, all-night cafes and cleaning crews, banks and post offices and all manner of vending machines, laboratories and operating rooms, delivery suites and mortuaries. They're not just twenty-four–hour places, they're townships.

And it's in these townships that we human beings get sick and well, birth and die. You find newborns and centenarians, the prematurely old and those with a new lease on life. Here are the over- and underweight, the addicted and abused, the halt and the lame, the pray-ers and prayed for, the healers and healees. Workers of every skill and color play their part in a hospital's dramas: high tragedy and soap opera, horror movie and high farce. You'll find doctors rubbing shoulders with repair men, nurses with lab techs, social workers with cleaning crews.

But despite all these life-and-death dramas—the miraculous recoveries and breakthroughs beloved by our media—most illness today comes on slowly and chronically. Perhaps this has been the case with you. These are the ailments of our Western civilization— legacies of stress-filled lifestyles and fast-food eating habits. They're rarely seen in indigenous cultures: high blood pressure, arthritis, osteoporosis, chronic backache and headache, cancer, cardiovascular and cerebrovascular disease, depression, anxiety and insomnia, hyperactivity and Alzheimer's disease. Each affects millions of us Americans, and costs billions in quick-fix treatments, as well as lost work and school time. Together they add up to a trillion dollars—the latest annual budget for American health care.

It's abundantly clear that hospitals and other places of health care need something more to set beside the medical science that is trying to stem this tide of illness: something that will make you really *feel better*, healthier in every way—not just in body but in mind and spirit too. This is what art and art-making offer: I'll show you how.

A Brief History

First though, I'm going to fill in a little background. Doctors until recently thought every illness was totally understandable, once we knew enough about your anatomy, physiology, and biochemistry. Your illness was also something quite beyond your control, either to prevent in the first place or do anything about once you were stuck with it.

This idea of illness was born 400 years ago with a couple of European philosophers, Francis Bacon and Rene Descartes (of "I think, therefore I am" fame). Bacon called science the "virile son" dominating Mother Nature as his slave, while Descartes was busy divorcing mind and spirit totally from body (the "Cartesian split"). Then along came another nonphysician, Isaac Newton, to expand these ideas. He saw us as machines, each bit reducible to minute constituents. Doctors bought into these ideas. From then on medicine occupied itself solely with scientifically measurable matters. Art—along with imagery, dreams, intuition, and spirituality—was no longer its concern. For every disease a custom-made remedy would be invented. Illness was the mortal enemy, hospitals battlefields where war was waged. Death, being the final failure, wasn't even talked about. The focus was on your individual organs in disorder, which is why we have so many medical specialties: cardiology, neurology, nephrology, oncology, and so on. It's not that specialists don't do life-saving work in the service of people with complicated ailments. It's just that the *total health* of your body, mind, and spirit has been sidelined. This is where art comes in.

Holism: Broadening the Scope

Today everyone can share in the care of their own health. Gone are the days of "paternalism," with doctors treating their passive and obedient patients like so many children, carrying out their tests and treatments with scant explanation. The Internet and lay publications are leveling the playing field. With a few resources you can find out all you want to know about your medical problem before you ever see a doctor. This is creating a healthy new environment of patient-doctor partnership.

A good example is the growing use of unconventional medicine by almost half our population, mostly for those chronic conditions I've mentioned that orthodox medicine isn't good at treating, let alone preventing. Up until recently most people took these remedies without telling their doctors, because they were frightened of their disapproval. This made for a big communication gap. But this state of affairs is changing, because both doctors and patients are realizing they're in partnership together. The reason why this is such an important and welcome shift in our approach to health is that the healing arts have stood the test of time. Many have been the medical mainstay of every traditional culture—from Africa and Australasia to Asia and the Americas—since prehistory. And these indigenous peoples never distinguished between healing and creative art. We now know that whether it's meditation or music, tai chi or dance, these therapies all call on the same physiological and biochemical pathways within you that work to enhance your overall health.

These new-but-old forms of self-care people are turning to today are usually called alternative or complementary medicine. A better word is *holistic,* because it embraces every aspect of health—physical, mental, spiritual, social, environmental. Your heart or liver or kidneys don't walk into your doctor's office asking to be "fixed." They come contained within your body, mind, and spirit—that of a well-informed or hopeful or frightened or denying human being. You bring with you your family and your work and your lifetime's habits, which you may or may not be willing or able to change. In short, you bring the story of your life. What holistic health care offers is a blend of science with art: a healthy doctor-patient relationship, patient education and responsibility, and all the arts of care and self-care, including the healing power of love, hope, and humor.

How to Use This Book

So read on, and give yourself the chance to be an artist again. And in doing so, prescribe for yourself (with a little guidance from me) the self-healing medicine of picture-making and poem-making, of dance and song and "acting the fool." In the process you'll have a thoroughly good time. But this is no trivial undertaking. The goal is not just to provide a temporary lift when you're feeling down. This book sets out to create lasting changes in your life—in how you deal with any illness or disability that you or a loved one may suffer from. One thing is certain: Illness is going to happen to each of us, if it hasn't already. This book will furnish you with some self-help tools that don't wear out.

You'll find many exercises that give you hands-on experience and practice in art-making of every kind. Some are easier than others. Some you can return to often, or use as an ongoing activity. Most you'll need companions for, either family members or friends, or people experiencing the same kind of life issues or problems as you. If you're in a hospital reading this book, or like most of us you're a very busy person, you may well find you're interrupted while doing these exercises. This is fine, because they're designed to come back to as often as you like. You may also find ways to weave many into your daily routine. You'll also find stories with a teaching purpose, about people who've had major illnesses or other life challenges to meet, which will I hope serve as an inspiration and example to you.

I'll describe later all the resources you'll need. They're neither numerous nor expensive. For the moment you'll simply need two or three sizeable workbooks. I use those sturdy ones with ring binders you can buy at any drug or stationery store. Make sure they're the sort you like, because they're going to be your friends and companions throughout your reading, and I hope beyond. The reason I suggest getting more than one is that, as well as doing exercises in your workbook, you'll be keeping a regular art sketchbook, as you'll find out in chapter 4, as well as a journal, which I'll describe in chapter 5. You may decide to use the same book for all these purposes, though, so that exercises, artwork, and journaling weave in and out.

You'll need three or four pens, of your very favorite kind. Again, I want you to make sure you enjoy picking them up and working with them. I suggest you get several because, if they're anything like mine, they'll do disappearing tricks on you when you need them most. And you certainly don't want to use up all your creative energies on a wild-goose chase just as you're ready to get down to your vital work of self-expression. I also suggest you buy your pens in different colors—say, blue, black, red, green, and even violet—because your first two lessons in being an artist once more are to love your art-making tools, and to bring to them as much variety as you can. While you're picking out your pens, pick up a set of assorted colored pencils too, for variety, together with a pencil sharpener and eraser.

Okay, that's all you'll need for the moment. Now for some creative self-expression . . .

1

Thriving, Not Just Surviving: Creative Self-Expression Can Help

Never never never under any circumstances face facts!
—Ruth Gordon

The Meanings of Art

The word *art* has lots of meanings. What comes to mind for you? You may at once picture an art museum with old-fashioned portraits or pastoral scenes in gilt-edged frames, or a Soho art gallery with colorful but unintelligible paintings on each wall, all at outrageous prices.

Perhaps you broadened your thinking to the performance arts—classical ballet, Shakespearean plays, and Wagnerian opera. You may have thought about the more everyday offerings of radio, TV, and film. Seen any good movies lately? Perhaps you're listening to music on your radio right now. There are very few people in this country who don't have access to a TV, catering as it does to everyone's taste in stories, drama, tragedy, and farce. Do you know any hospitals that don't have one hanging over the foot of every bed? Is this art, do you think?

Then there are those so-called literary arts. Have you read any good books lately—or listened to one on tape? What about poetry—have you noticed there's a lot of it around nowadays? You may have chosen to avoid it, and hated it with a passion, ever since you had to learn poems by rote at school.

A Broader Definition

But do you notice a common theme to these examples? They all refer to *professionals*—painters and writers and actors and musicians who believe they have the talent to make a living at it, or at least sell some of their work to the public. And of course they're all at the mercy of those judging them—directors, gallery owners, critics, us— their viewers and readers and listeners. It's all about making these judgments on whether one piece of artwork is any better than another. This is the legacy of the competitive get-ahead world we've grown up in. We've been taught to ask not "Is it art?" but "How *good* is it? How talented is the artist? Which one will make it—become fashionable, draw in the crowds, sell a million copies, or even be worth investing in?"

Let's try broadening this term "art" a bit. What about you? Have you picked up a paintbrush since primary school? Do you doodle little drawings when you're on the phone? Do you sing Christmas carols or rock-and-roll songs in the shower? Do you do *any* kind of dancing? Come on—don't you even tap your feet to the rhythm of the radio? What about playing a musical instrument? Have you ever tried? Have you shared any stories lately, or perhaps written some heartfelt lines in a letter to a friend, or to yourself in your journal? Haven't you ever memorized a joke so you could tell it to get the best laugh?

Even if the answer is a resounding "No!" to every one of these examples, just cast your mind back to your childhood for a moment. Were there any of these things that you *didn't* do in those days?

Webster's defines art as "creative work generally . . . the making and doing of things that have form and beauty . . ." It doesn't say anything about doing it *well*. Beauty is in the eye of the beholder, right? If you take away the judgment for a moment (I know, not an easy thing to do), then we're every one of us artists, creators, from the moment of our births. We all *make things up*.

Story: Thanksgiving

On Thanksgiving Eve, the patients and their caregivers gathered for the weekly workshop at Charlie's Corner, the hospital cancer unit's family room. The patients, most of them middle-aged and a long way from home, trailed their IV poles behind them. The volunteers settled them in rockers and armchairs.

Today was Storytelling Hour. Don, the hospice chaplain, led off with a memory from his childhood about sugar-cane grinding, how his farmer-uncle Tom always let the mule pulling the tractor get in a good slurp at the cane syrup before it was carted off to the vats for boiling. Bob, a chatty Florida "cracker," told a tale of family reunions at trestle tables, set up outside the house and groaning with food, and how one time he got so sick he was stuck in bed for the celebration. Liza told a family joke that was trotted out every Thanksgiving about her toddler sister sticking a bit of chicken up her nose that wasn't found for a week.

The stories flowed back and forth—mostly funny, often poignant, all warm and cheering. For a while cancer and chemotherapy were forgotten as the room took on the true feeling of what indeed it was: a family room at holiday time. Finally, Don told the story of the pilgrims giving thanks in early-1600s Massachusetts, despite half their number having died that first terrible year, since they'd clambered down the Mayflower Steps at Plymouth Ho! Harbor.

Then it was time for the singalong. The old favorites were trotted out, after Don had instructed this impromptu choir that "harmonizing is just singing any note no one else is on." After a practice verse or two of "America the Beautiful," the group decided to move on to the nurses' station and serenade the staff. After all, they were stuck here for the holiday too. Everyone shuffled their way from the family room to the nurses' station, forming themselves into a semicircle with Don as choirmaster. As the ragged voices of five patients and five volunteers carried through the ward, there was lots of laughter, not a few tears, and thanksgiving on all sides.

Art as Care

Hold it in your mind for a moment, this scene on the cancer ward. Let's think a bit about what was going on here. Because they were far from being professionals, I venture *artist* is the last word those patients would have used to describe themselves, even *after* they'd given their very first choral performance. Every one of them had been reluctant to take the floor and become storytellers, until Don gave them permission with his gentle coaxing. And the idea of singing, of being part of a choir, at first brought loud protests. But once they got into it, began thinking up all those old favorites, they soon realized that no one else was hitting, let alone holding, their notes too well either. And how quickly they all caught on to the idea of offering a musical thanksgiving gift to their nurses. They wouldn't have missed that for the world.

So for a few minutes the caregivers of these seriously ill patients were themselves on the receiving end of loving care—in the form of art—from the very ones they were there to serve. And the patients, with their shared stories and their off-key singing, had perhaps taken another step forward in their healing journey, for themselves and for each other.

Which brings us to the other accepted meaning of the word *art:* that of giving loving care and service to each other, to anyone in need. Put another way, this is what is meant by the art of caring and skilled service to the sick, the disabled, and the dying, young and old. It's just as vital a component of health care as the last hundred years of medical scientific progress. Just as in education the arts are often contrasted with the sciences, so in health care art and science are seen as opposites. Actually of course they're complements, and of equal importance, because they're both indispensable. This is a self-help book that will teach you practical ways to use art-making in all its wonderful guises for your greater health and happiness. The word art, used in this way, is really an analogy for devoting your whole life, in sickness and in health, to living a healthy life, together with your family and friends, colleagues and acquaintances—all the time.

Exercise: Reclaim the Artist Within!

I talked in the introduction about how as a young child you were freely urged by your parents and early teachers to make art of all kinds. It was only later, when you felt that pressure to compete and get ahead, that you got the message that you must put those idle pursuits behind you—that you were having altogether too much fun!

Well, now's the chance to have fun once more. You're going to do an easy exercise in art-making: making pictures, both visual and verbal. The sole purpose is for you to find out just how simple and fun it is to make art. I'm not concerned right now with proving anything to you about its healing effects. I just want you to loosen up, and lighten up, and rediscover that you can both draw and write creatively.

This will be your very first entry in your workbook. We'll start with visual art. Open up your book and place it to one side, so it's just out of your sight when you gaze straight ahead. Put it on your right if you're right-handed, and to your left if you're a lefty. Now choose your favorite pen (blue or red or green) and lay it on the open page. Next, close your eyes and take two or three deep, slow letting-down breaths. Fill your lungs right up each time. Open your eyes, and look straight in front of you at what lies within your range of vision. Don't look around, just more or less straight ahead.

Let your eyes light on any object that pleases you. Make it an object of finite size, not too big—not for example the whole wall opposite you. It could be a flower in a vase, a slipper or a sneaker, or your companion's hand or face. Now slowly follow the contours of this object with your eyes—all its ins and outs. Do this a couple of times, and then, while your eyes are still traveling, pick up your pen and start to let it follow the exact same directions as your eyes, as close as you can, on the open page. Try hard not to look over at your drawing. Let yourself relax into it, softening your hand on the page, moving it always in the same contours as your eyes.

Gradually pick up the pace a bit. Keep going for two or three minutes, then stop and look over at your handiwork. Well, did anything terrible happen? Or does your drawing look pretty much like the object you were looking at? Okay. Move your pen and your hand down the page to some blank space. Or turn to a new page. Now bring your eyes back to the object, and begin the exercise of following its contours all over again. Start your hand moving across the page once more, resisting any temptation to look at what you're doing. Slow down a bit, taking more time with the outline of your object. Relax into it, relishing the feeling of your pen on the paper, recreating the image. Try to keep going until you're unaware of concentrating on the task—or until the pull is too strong for you to resist looking over at what you've created.

You can repeat this exercise as often as you like, changing the objects of your attention. But usually three or four times is enough to show you just how easy it is to be a visual artist, and to produce without effort a lifelike image of the object that caught your fancy. Now, most importantly—pause to give yourself some lavish praise for your work of art—you artist, you! Before moving on, make sure you've entered the date, including the day of the week and time of day. It's a good habit also to sign your work, adding a note about where you are right now, as a reminder for the future. If you want to comment on how you're feeling, go right ahead and be my guest! This is an excellent habit to get into, and will be fun to review at a later time.

Exercise: Reclaim the Writer Within!

You'll be doing a lot more exercises in picture-making in chapter 4, and learning how you can use many art materials with the greatest of ease. This was a warm-up to get you started. Right now you're going to try your hand at some *creative writing*. Creative writing is anything that isn't technical, scientific, or a shopping list. For the purposes of this book, you might call it self-help writing. You'll do a lot of similar exercises in chapter 5, but for now I just want to get you limbered up.

Let's carry on from the drawing exercise. Take a look at the several pictures you made of the commonplace object that caught your fancy. Perhaps it was a stray sock, or the patterned eiderdown comforter on your bed, or something on the tray of leftover breakfast things. What does this object say to you? Take a trip down memory lane. What memories do you have of socks or beds or breakfasts that you've known?

Close your eyes and breathe easily. Let your mind run on. Allow yourself to recall occasions from your childhood—getting ready for school, say. Are they good or sad memories? Where were you? What was the time of year? Pick up your pen and start writing down whatever comes into your mind.

Try to get your very first thought down on the page; don't block it. Trust your right brain to throw up memories that are worth recalling and recording. Just keep your hand moving, without judgment. Feel the pen in your hand, watch it gliding across the page. Enjoy the gentle sensation, but don't focus on the words coming up and forth. Have a good time with whatever it is you're thinking of, filling in the blanks with your imagination if you lose some details. But do go for the details: Who was with you? How old were you? What were you wearing? Who was doing all the talking? How did you feel about them? How did you feel about yourself? Why do you think that particular memory came up right now?

And so on ... keep writing for about ten minutes, until you have three or four paragraphs. If possible, don't pause for more than a moment, and don't let your present circumstances intrude. Most of all, don't give an ounce of legroom to your *inner critic*. Whatever you write down is absolutely fine. It all comes from your authentic self: the writer within you. If you feel the urge, put in some strong language—some swear words if they help you express the real you. Remember, this is just for your eyes and ears, unless of course you ever choose to share it with anyone else.

Memories of Illness

I hope you enjoyed uncovering once more the instinctive writer within you. It wasn't so hard, was it? Remember to sign and date your work, including the time of day, and say a word or two about your present circumstances and feelings.

You may have enjoyed writing about a joyful memory from your earlier life. Or something may have surfaced that was sad or hard to remember. If so, I hope you didn't block it out and move on to easier things. Many people who have a present ailment or affliction to deal with find themselves reminded of earlier occasions when they were ill or had to go to the hospital, perhaps for an operation or something similar. This next exercise will help you focus in a little more detail on your past, or present, experience of illness, or your visit to the hospital for whatever reason. It will help you get a sense of what to look for, so you can tell if your hospital or other place of care is giving enough attention to the art as well as the science of medicine. All you'll need is your workbook for writing down your story. There may be more than one version of it, though, because everyone's life is made up of many interweaving stories.

Exercise: A Hospital Visit

Think about the last time you were in a hospital. Perhaps you're an inpatient right now, reading this book from your hospital bed, or you might be in an outpatient clinic keeping your regular appointment. Maybe you've been visiting a friend or a family member who is sick. Perhaps your doctor wanted a second opinion on a bothersome symptom that you'd had for a while. You might have needed surgery (not, I hope, for a serious problem).

Let your mind dwell on the familiar hospital scenes before your eyes. Take a look around, or picture a recent scene in your mind's eye. How was it—or is it? Terrifying or tedious? Daunting or downright miserable? Tragic, or was there some light relief? Perhaps the surroundings were depressing—or were there some uplifting features? The staff may be helpful, caring people, or maybe everyone is too rushed to listen to you. Is everything bustle and noise, or have you managed to find a place of quiet and repose? There may be art on the walls. Is there relaxing music to listen to in the hallways and corridors? Are there even live plants anywhere to help keep you in touch with the outside world? How about the signs—the "wayfinders"? Are they easy, even pleasing, to read? Are the meals nutritious and prepared with care, or are they mostly overcooked and fattening fast food?

Jot down these observations, and especially your feelings about them, in your workbook. Note the impressions that all these images leave on you, whether they're positive or negative. Try creating a credit/debit sheet in your workbook, with the nurturing and artful things in the left-hand column and the dull and dismal items on the right, something like this:

Positive	Negative
Nice people	Crazy maze of a place
Not too noisy	Everyone in a hurry
Pictures on the walls	Dull colors, no pictures
Music in the waiting room	Long dark corridors

... and so on.

Aesthetic Environments

Art in all its many manifestations has a vital role to play in our hospitals and other places of healing, especially for those who have to make repeated clinic visits or spend long periods of time as an inpatient. If you have a chronic illness like diabetes or high blood pressure or arthritis, believe me, you're far from alone. Estimates put the figure for the number of people in this country suffering from chronic illnesses and disabilities at over 100 million—not far off half our U.S. population. It's safe to assume that most of the rest of the population are in some way affected by this, often by being involved in their care, either as family, friends, or professional caregivers.

Evidence from a lot of research I'll go over with you later confirms the value to your health of an aesthetically pleasing environment. So as a consumer of health care you have the right to expect this aspect to receive plenty of attention, and indeed funding. You have a right to quiet and secluded surroundings, or ones where there is calming music available. You have a right to find around you relaxing or inspiring pictures, with someone thinking about the impact on you of the colors of the walls and ceilings. You have a right to plenty of natural light, with real live plants to keep you in touch with the outside. These things have significant effects on your overall health. I'm glad to report that many hospitals are beginning to recognize this and budget accordingly.

Exercise: Art in Hospitals

This simple exercise goes a bit further, making you the definitive judge of your hospital's attention to all aspects of art and aesthetics. The goal is to give you a measure of how *healthy* your hospital is, in a holistic sense. We'll come back to that word *holistic* later. For the moment, think of it as referring to your whole health: of your body, mind, and spirit, and of both you as an individual and of your community.

Think once more about your last hospital visit, or focus on your current day if you're spending it in one. I want you to grade your experience from 0 to 4 under the categories I've listed in the table on the next page. Use the following scale: 0 means very negative, 1 negative, 2 neutral, 3 positive, 4 very positive. You can circle them in pencil in the book or, even better, use your workbook to reproduce the exercise. Notice that I've chosen these items as having nothing directly to do with the specific reason for your hospital visit. The evidence is that the higher your score on this exercise, the more beneficial to your *overall* health your trip to the hospital is likely to be or have been. I've inserted some prompts, but you can think up other aspects of your experience that might affect your score.

TOTAL SCORE: _____ (Max = 76)

Less than 20 = Get me outta here!

20–40 = Ho hum!

40–60 = They're trying!

Over 60 = A healing place!

If you scored over 60 points, your recent or current hospital experience has been a pretty positive one. The administrators and caregivers are putting some emphasis on aesthetics and other aspects of design that contribute to making it a healing place. They're thinking about *you* as a whole person, not just about your illness and its treatment. You probably won't mind a return visit. You may well feel that your trip or your stay is helping you be healthier in mind and spirit, as well as physically. If you scored 40 to 60, you can give your caregivers and hospital administrators credit for trying. They may well be open to some suggestions from you as to other ways they can make a difference. If you scored 20 to 40, there is at least a glimmer of hope. See if you can spot any new healing efforts in the environment at your next visit. If you scored under 20, you probably felt or feel mostly incarcerated and uncared for during your hospital visit. The *art* of healing is not getting much attention.

Science and Art as Partners

Until recently, medical science was threatening to displace healing art altogether. But the pendulum's swinging back. We're waking to the truth that most illnesses, even the chronic and incurable ones, can be prevented from worsening when caregivers attend to you as a whole person, and to the community of which you're a part. Most chronic illness could in fact be prevented altogether if our society had an overall healthy lifestyle in the first place. Even if you do have an

	0	1	2	3	4
SIGHTS					
Approaches	Ugly, daunting	Dull, colorless	Neutral	Fresh, colorful	Beautiful
Signage	Ugly, daunting	Dull, colorless	Neutral	Fresh, colorful	Beautiful
Light	Dark or glaring	No outside light	Neutral	Thoughtful	Harmonious
Walls	Bare, dirty	Functional	Neutral	Color, art	Plenty of art
Rooms	Bare, dirty	Functional	Neutral	Color, art	Plenty of art
Floors & Ceilings	Ugly, dirty	Functional	Neutral	Comfy, calm	Harmonious
SOUNDS					
Main areas	Turbulent	Noisy	Neutral	Mostly quiet	Restful
Clinic areas	Turbulent	Noisy	Neutral	Mostly quiet	Restful
Wards	Turbulent	Noisy	Neutral	Mostly quiet	Restful
Rooms	Turbulent	Noisy	Neutral	Mostly quiet	Restful
ATMOSPHERE					
Main areas	Smelly, cold	Tolerable	Neutral	Fresh, warm	Harmonious
Clinic areas	Smelly, cold	Tolerable	Neutral	Fresh, warm	Harmonious
Wards	Smelly, cold	Tolerable	Neutral	Fresh, warm	Harmonious
Rooms	Smelly, cold	Tolerable	Neutral	Fresh, warm	Harmonious
PEOPLE					
Staff	Unhappy, cold	Burdened	Neutral	Happy, warm	Harmonious
Patients	Miserable	Burdened	Neutral	Content	Harmonious
Others	Miserable	Burdened	Neutral	Content	Harmonious
EATING AREAS					
Food	Inedible	Pretty bad	Neutral	Good	Healthy, tasty
Surroundings	Ugly	Pretty bad	Neutral	Artful	Harmonious

established illness already—one doctors term incurable—there are many things you can do for yourself to live a fuller, happier life. Art-making is one of them.

Even if your doctor hasn't put much stress on this aspect of your care, the medical profession as a whole is coming to recognize that health care is science and art in equal part. They're not opposites. Each one calls for imagination and creativity, as well as the courage to plunge into the unknown. Each calls on the intuitive and inventive part of our human intelligence. Scientists, like artists, play around with the variables that our universe offers—particles and mole-cules and color and light—to make some order and beauty out of them. But in the end the true art of health care should enable you to live the very healthiest and happiest life you can, whatever your circumstances.

Symptoms and Symbols

Are you convinced yet of the value of rekindling your creativity, in the face of whatever illness or disability you may have? While doc-tors and nurses struggle with merging science and art in their work, perhaps you the patient find these new-but-old ideas confusing, even frightening. You may be wondering how this mix can best work for you, the person on the receiving end of health care. It helps to remember too that every one of us is going to be on the receiving end sometime. None of us is excluded from meeting illness, and ulti-mately death, face to face.

What art can offer in these circumstances is a new way of understanding illness and coming to terms with it. It can lead you to new ways of being healthy even when you have a life-limiting illness. Art can give you tools to use that don't require a medical degree or deep scientific knowledge. You may have already found that, when life lays a bad break on you, you deal with it best when you can make sense of it, and derive some meaning from your experience. So it is with illness and disability. You may wonder why you—or any of us—got ill in the first place. You may ask yourself (and everyone else), "Why me? Why now? Why this illness?" We probably all have questions like this at one time or another. Art will help you see the common link between the outward symptoms and signs that first brought your illness to your attention and the inner symbols it repre-sents for your mind and spirit.

Story: Danny and Rose

I remember my conversations with the mother of a ten-year-old boy with a rare, hard-to-treat form of cancer. I'll call her Rose. Her son—Danny, I'll call him—was able to stay home and come to my clinic for much of his treatment. But as time went on he needed more frequent hospital stays.

At first Rose was angry and demanding, questioning my decisions and criticizing the nurses during procedures. She'd ask several people the same question, as though testing us for consistency. The resident doctors avoided going into Danny's room. Then as time went on, even though Danny's condition was getting worse, a change came over Rose. Most striking was the emergence of her sense of humor. The change in atmosphere was immeasurable. From dreading to be assigned to Danny's care, the nurses and pediatric resident doctors came to welcome the chance to sit and chat with Rose and her dying son.

Toward the end Danny needed a tracheostomy (a tube inserted into his windpipe to assist his breathing). He remained fully conscious though, talking in a hoarse croak by covering the opening with his hand. Rose urged him to take pride in his excellent Donald Duck imitations. It became a frequent game as to who—Danny or Rose—was going to do the suctioning needed to keep his airway clear and get enough oxygen. At first frustrated by his resistance to her help, Rose finally became proud of her son's independence. When it got hard to stop the buildup of phlegm and repeated attempts had to be made, Danny would "quack" at his mother: "Get your own (blank blank) tracheostomy," at which point she would perform a pantomime of suctioning herself.

A couple of days before he died I was sitting on his bed while he was sleeping. I asked Rose why she thought this tragedy had been visited on her and Danny. Did it *mean*—or symbolize—anything to her? I probed a little about her change of attitude toward us.

"I know, I bet you dreaded seeing me coming," she said. "It's just that for the longest time I couldn't make any sense of it. Why me, God? What have I ever done to deserve this?" She looked down at Danny peacefully asleep. "One day I took a look at him, saw how frail he was becoming, how much he was hurting, but how he never stopped being cheerful, looking on the bright side. He was the sick one, yet he was always trying to perk me up.

"I suddenly thought: Well, no one's answering my prayers for an explanation to all this, so maybe I'd better just settle down and make the best of it. That was when I remembered myself at ten, how I was always the joker in the family and among my friends. I suddenly saw how serious I'd become. Well, it was time to lighten up, for his sake. So right then I told him: 'Thanks, Danny, for giving me back my sense of humor!'"

Stories and Meanings

So, for Rose, Danny's illness, though of course enormously tragic, had at least one benefit. Even, or perhaps especially, in his advanced state, Danny reawoke in her the lost joy of her childhood ways. He gave her back her art—that of humor—something she'd long put aside, but something at which she'd obviously been a pretty good artist. This gave meaning, or symbolism, to what had happened to Danny and herself.

People with serious illnesses and their families want to "know" why it's happened to them. You may have had this experience. It's not so much a scientific answer you're looking for, but more a philosophical one—not strictly rational in the usual sense of the word. The words "symbol" and "symptom" have a common origin: that of things being thrown together. From this they've come to mean the outward signs to us of something hidden from our conscious awareness.

In a very real sense, the symptoms you develop when an illness or disability affects you are symbolic of what that illness *means* to you. Your body tells you what you need to hear, no matter how often you try to silence it. If you or a loved one are ill, you may have tried to create a story to explain it, one that has pieces of your own life and those of your family woven into its fabric. You may not even be aware of creating this story until you reflect on it.

Studies of this common practice have shown that the symbolism people use is sometimes punishing. But more often it frees you from blame and helps lighten your suffering. With a little space to cry and rage if you choose to, and finally to talk and reflect on your story, you'll often find an explanation coming along that will serve to give you acceptance, even forgiveness if need be. This acceptance will in turn bring emotional and even physical relief—peace of mind, body, and spirit.

The Stories of our Lives

Physician-philosopher Howard Brody talks in his book *Stories of Sickness* (1987) about how we're each of us the stories of our lives. If you can see the experience of your sickness as a meaningful story, it will help ease the suffering you may be feeling. You make use of this art whenever you listen to another or they listen to you, and you can reflect on what the meaning of an illness might be. Research confirms the healing value of telling your stories. This is what lies at the heart of all psychotherapy.

Someone once said illness is nature's way of slowing you down. It certainly can offer you this chance to take some time for yourself, so you can delve a little deeper into the meanings of things, and the purpose of your life. The universe surely has its reasons for everything, unless you see yourself as some kind of human billiard ball—cannonballing off other balls at the whim of the gods until you get buried in some random pocket or other. At the end of his life, Albert Einstein said: "The most important question all of us must answer is whether the universe is a friendly place or not." I think our universe is a friendly and loving place for us to inhabit together, if you let it be.

No amount of logical thinking or medical science, though, is going to help you explain why *this* illness affected *you* at *this time*. John Keats, who graduated as a doctor from London University 150 years before me, said toward the end of his short life as one of the greatest poets ever: "I am certain of nothing but the holiness of the heart's affections, and the truth of the imagination." This is the imaginative and intuitive truth that art offers. There's no better time than when you're ill to uncover this side of the truth, so it can add to the incomplete facts medical science gives you.

Exercise: Telling Your Story

This exercise will show you something about how you think about illness, how you explain it, what purposes it might serve, and some of your feelings about being sick. It may help you equate the outward signs of your illness with symbols, or psychic explanations for illness in your life. This is the art of story-telling. All you'll need is your workbook, a pen or pencil, and twenty minutes of uninterrupted time.

Cast your mind back to a time when you were sick. If you're suffering from an illness or disability right now, use it for this exercise. You're going to write a story of your experience as if you were telling it to your best friend, or to your doctor or nurse. But make it a *story*, not a list of dates and facts and past treatments (the sort of thing you've probably supplied many times when giving the history of your illness and its symptoms). Like all the best stories, it needs a beginning, a middle, and an end. Here are a few questions to ask yourself to get going:

- When do you think this illness first took up occupancy inside you?
- Who else is involved?
- Why do you think it picked you out of the pack?
- Does it remind you of anything that happened to you in your past?

- If your illness could talk to you, what do you think it would say?
- What do you want to tell it in return?
- If your illness was a play, what kind of play would it be? A tragedy, a whodunit thriller, or a farce?
- What are the worst things about it?
- Is your life different in any way since your illness?
- Is there anything at all good you can say about the situation?
- What have you learned, if anything, from being sick?
- Has your illness served any purpose? For you or anyone else?

Got the idea? I expect you can come up with similar or quite different questions about your personal experience of illness or disability. Reflect on your questions, writing a sentence or two in answer to each. Out of these reflections perhaps you can weave a story about your recent journey through life. When you've put something down in answer to each, go back and add to them wherever you feel inclined. Be as fanciful as you like—it's *your* story.

Okay, finish up when you're ready. I hope it's been helpful to exercise your story-teller's art and apply it to your own situation. You can return to your tale any time you like. I'll be inviting you to do so during the course of your reading this book. As you learn other ways of expressing yourself artistically, you may want to draw pictures, write a poem, even compose a short play or song about your life right now. You'll learn more in this book about *restoring yourself by restorying yourself.*

Studies Support Support Groups

Meanwhile, whatever your state of health or illness may be, I assure you *sister art* is taking her rightful place once more beside *brother science* in the service of people in sickness and in health. The art of nurturing care is alive and well, as in the healing effects of support groups. Dr. David Spiegel, a psychiatrist at Stanford University, carried out a study ten years ago with women with breast cancer (1989). He found that those whose treatment included a peer-support group lived twice as long as those who received standard medical care. An AIDS support group in Los Angeles took on an even more creative project—writing and producing its own play about living with AIDS.

Cardiologist Dean Ornish, in his book *Love and Survival* (1998), documents many other studies of support groups for patients with heart disease. The strength and extent of your social networks can have a vital effect on lowering your risk of further heart attacks; this is preventive medicine at its best. These studies show how much all of us need each other to help maintain healthy bodies, minds, and spirits. Doctors and psychologists are starting to accept the importance of partnership, as well as a sense of personal control over your life. Instead of asking: "What disease does this patient have?", medicine is finally reframing it as: "Who's the patient who has this disease?"

⟋ *Exercise: Building Support*

So art, as I'm offering it to you, is a healing tool that is best used in the company of others. I won't be urging you to go off into some isolated attic to create great works of genius—quite the reverse. Art-making is a way to bring together people like yourself over a common interest, breaking down the artificial but often strong barriers between people in our society. These barriers can be a real threat to your health and longevity.

This exercise will help you identify areas of interest or experience you share with others, so you can figure out how to bring together a group of people for mutual support and health benefits. Perhaps you're already part of such a group. But this isn't at all the same thing as a bunch of men going to the ball game, or a group of women friends taking off on a shopping spree. Its focus is social connectedness for its healing benefits. Fifteen to twenty minutes should give you plenty of time for this exercise, and you can always come back to it. I've offered some suggestions to get you started.

The things I'd want to get from such a support group are:

- Specific information and helpful reading

- A chance to talk about my illness and listen to others talk about theirs

- A chance to meet with similar folk in a problem-solving setting

- A time to cheer myself up and forget my troubles

- Activities or a project we can work on together

- Help with changing my unhealthy behaviors

- Specific healing tools for myself and others

- Help with getting the word out to others about our specific health needs

- Other

To get such a group started I'll need:

- To find others with similar issues or problems
  (List possible names)

- To find a place and time to meet
  (List possible places and frequencies)

- To get help from a health professional
  (List possible names)

- To find someone else to share the organizing work
  (List possible names)

- To brainstorm topics for discussion
  (List possible topics)

- To get started, my next steps will be:
  (List your tasks as precisely as you can)
  (Draw up definite deadlines for yourself)

With these goals and deadlines you've made for yourself, you've taken a big step toward building the kind of support in which art-making activities fit perfectly.

2

Artful Care: Helping Yourself and Others

Never go to a doctor whose office plants have died.

—Erma Bombeck

Taking Charge of Your Health

Who is really in charge of your health? Who decides what's best for you? Is it you—or your caregivers? What if you disagree? How often is the right thing to do clear-cut from *all* viewpoints? If you or a family member have a serious or chronic illness, you've probably wrestled with these sorts of questions, consciously or unconsciously. Many people feel they're not really in charge, that their doctors don't give them the chance to be fully involved, to be partners together.

The reason seems to be health care's narrow focus. Doctors are trained to be lifesavers at all costs, with science often overruling art. As our society's life expectancy gets longer and longer, some doctors even imagine they can keep people alive indefinitely. With enough spare-part surgery, genetic engineering, and an ever-growing menu of drugs, it can get hard for doctors to practice caring art side by side with curing science. This is where your rights as a patient come in. It's vital that you build a partnership between you and your doctor— one that gives you an equal share in deciding what's best for you in any given situation.

Story: Ed My Student-Teacher

I had a patient I'll call Ed. He'd been an easy bruiser all his life. A small cut when he was shaving just wouldn't stop bleeding. He knew to use soft toothbrushes or his gums would bleed too. The doctors who'd seen him before had run a battery of tests to pinpoint most conditions that cause excessive bleeding, like hemophilia. They'd all been normal. The additional tests I could think of were just as unrevealing. I was tempted to put his symptoms down to a "variation of the norm," and metaphorically pat him on the back.

My reassurances didn't satisfy Ed. He was sure he had some funny condition I wasn't putting my finger on. He'd done some reading about family bleeding problems, and researched his own extended family. He found out that both a great-uncle and a second cousin had had similar troubles. Like most students he was a computer whiz. On his next visit he arrived with a pile of printouts: the soup-to-nuts of bleeding disorders. He pointed out one or two rare conditions and asked me point-blank if I'd tested for them. I had to admit I hadn't. You may have guessed it: Ed had a rare inherited condition later identified in the other two men in his family. It was just as well he pushed me to make the diagnosis because a few months later he needed major surgery, and we were able to give him his missing clotting factor ahead of time.

Placebo: I Will Please

Many studies support the benefits of taking some responsibility for dealing with your illness, as well as establishing a close relationship with your caregivers. It's important to have faith in each other. Just the act of a doctor taking your pulse can lessen your irregular heartbeats. Most medical treatments used a century ago had little scientific value, yet patients often did well and continued to seek help from their doctors. Any form of medical treatment will benefit you if you believe in it enough, as has been shown with sugar pills that relieve pain, bring down blood pressure, or fix an asthmatic wheeze.

This is very much the art of medicine, and doctors have long ago learned to put this *placebo* effect to good use. But it's equally certain that you can help your doctor and yourself. Develop an attitude of optimism and healthy expectation and you're more than likely to get what you expect. It's called a self-fulfilling prophecy. As I describe how art-making can benefit you, I'll remind you often of this simple truth, that belief in your own abilities and your capacity for self-healing will make all the difference to your ultimate health.

Story: Here's to Your Health!

My father was a general practitioner in the county of Devon in rural England in the 1930s, which were pre-penicillin days. Having very few specific treatments for what ailed these shepherds, thatchers, and blacksmiths, he served them all up with potions he dispensed himself—very visibly and with a lot of ceremony—from deep, square bottles labeled with names like *Camphora officianalis* and *Nux vomica*. They were perched for all to gaze upon, on high shelves lining the walls of his office—reminiscent of an eighteenth-century apothecary's shop.

All he insisted on was that these simple farmers and their wives, and even their children, quaff these placebos from narrow-stemmed wine glasses. His instruction about the particular container I'm sure contributed a major part to their beneficial effects; it seems his customers were well pleased with him and his potions.

Fifty years later this placebo (in Latin it means literally "I will please") effect is getting the recognition it deserves. It's no longer discounted as an inconvenience just because we don't fully understand how it works in your body. Even today doctors prescribe a huge compendium of medicines, many of them not proven by scientific studies to have any therapeutic effect. Yet patients get better from most ailments for which they seek medical help. It's this placebo of the loving and present intention of another who serves you, and whom you trust, that helps heal you from everything from asthma to angina, collywobbles to chicken pox.

It comes from several factors other than strictly medical ones, but most of all from your belief in the treatment and the strength of the partnership between giver and receiver. It can work in any situation where one person is trying to help another, like in a support group. Here's an easy exercise to illustrate this.

Exercise: Picturing Your Health

You can do this exercise by yourself, but it's fun to do with a friend or your support group. You'll need your workbook and colored pens or crayons. You're going to make a picture of a *totally healthy future you*. Whatever your current life circumstances, there's always room for improvement, right? So you're going to envision your total health and well-being. Then you're going to write a description of this person—the future you—depicting every part of yourself: your body, mind, and spirit, your social circumstances, and your relation to your environment. Then you're going to date it. In time you'll find out how good you are at self-fulfilling prophecies, how well you can make this placebo effect work for you.

So take up your workbook and turn to a fresh page. Get your multicolored crayons ready. Close your eyes and relax. Breathe deep and free, letting go a little more with each breath. When you're feeling calm and quiet, after maybe ten such breaths, let your imagination start to work. Start to envision yourself at some future time that is not too far distant. See yourself as the picture of health, whatever that looks like to you. It might mean physically vigorous and fit, alert and calm in your mind, full of wonder and delight at the joy of your life, with richly satisfying relationships, and so on.

When you're ready—meaning you have a clear image of yourself in front of you—open your eyes. Take up your box of crayons and select two or three colors that especially appeal to you. Start to draw the outline of your body's contours on the page. Now—this is very important. Just because you're depicting your ideal self doesn't mean that suddenly you've got to come up with a marvelous work of art. Nor do you have to use colors that exactly match your body and clothing. All you're trying to do is capture this image of yourself, so you can give yourself the gift of an ideal version to shoot for. You want something to look forward to, don't you? Let this be a depiction of just how you'd like every aspect of yourself to be.

You'll want to see yourself not only as sound in body, mind, and spirit, but in your ideal environment, and completely content with your lot in relation to those around you. These may be friends and loved ones, family and work colleagues. What are your future life circumstances? Put them there too. All you need is a representation of the most important parts. Pick out other crayons that give your picture even more power and vitality as you fill in the details. Don't hold back; for once give yourself a gift of just how you'd like your life to be.

When you're done (for the moment, because you can always come back to it), sign your name and add the date and place, as well as a sentence or two describing what you've depicted. Mostly, though, this is a visual image, so it doesn't need too many words. The crucial thing is that you believe in this picture of your ideal self you've created. This is the placebo—the "I will please"—at work on your behalf. If you believe enough in what you can do, then it can come to pass.

Exercise: Befriending Your Doctor

Now let's get some more support for you. This exercise is about friendship, and it may be especially helpful if you have a chronic illness and see your doctor quite often. I invite you to think about befriending her or him, getting to know as much about their life circumstances as they know about yours. In other words, I invite you to share your stories. By changing the usual context of this relationship, there's a good chance you'll find yourself feeling much more refreshed and happy. It's not essential that it's your doctor, but it would be good if it's someone who has some influence on what happens to you in relation to any illness or disability you may have. If your doctor seems standoffish or too busy to spend a few minutes of downtime with you, you might find this easier with one of your other caregivers in the clinic or on the ward—perhaps a nurse or a social worker, a ward clerk or a medical student if you're in a teaching hospital. Don't get discouraged, just quietly insist that you make one of your caregivers a new friend.

Try picturing this chosen person as if you'd met them at a party, or sat next to them on an airplane journey between New York and Seattle. You'll have to set it up a bit, tell them that next time they have a few minutes to spare you'd like to have a conversation with them. Tell them that just this once you'd like it to not be about your blood pressure or bowels. I've suggested a few topics you might cover, but you can add as many as you want. You might favor simple getting-to-know-you questions at first, moving on later to more philosophical issues that many health professionals think about a lot. It doesn't have to be forced. There are almost always clues around that tell you about people's lives outside of their work.

- Where were you raised? Do you have brothers and sisters? Are you married? Children?

- Do you have any pets? What kinds? What are their names? Who takes care of them?

- When did you decide to become a doctor/nurse/whatever? What made you decide? Why did you choose the kind of work you're in?

- How much time off do you get? What do you like to do with it? Where have you been on vacation recently?

- What are your favorite foods? TV shows? Movies? What kinds of books do you like to read?

- What do you think about the future of health care? What will the hospitals of tomorrow look like? What are we going to do about our national health care bill?

- Why do you think God invented illness? Why on earth can't we live forever, in perfect health?

And so on. Many caregivers—especially doctors—lead rather isolated lives, having been taught to keep a professional distance from their patients. The old-fashioned reason for this, that it will impair their judgment to get too close to a patient, has no basis in fact. The reverse is more likely true. Relaxing and sharing a bit of my own life with my patients has become a habit with me. I've found it helps me enjoy my "patient contact" time much more, with the result that I'm inclined to spend more time with them, and even to think more clearly when dealing with their health issues as they come up.

The Art of Togetherness

At the heart of healing is friendship and togetherness. Dr. Patch Adams—the clown doctor of *Gesundheit!* (1998) made famous by Robin Williams in the movie that bears Patch's name—has made a lifetime's healing habit of befriending total strangers, in airports or elevators or wherever. He honed this art of friendship as a student by spending endless hours dialing random telephone numbers and getting the stranger at the other end engaged in spontaneous and uproarious conversation. Now that takes the courage of your art-making convictions! From there on he's taken his art to 310 acres of West Virginia forest: the site of the first totally free and funny hospital. Togetherness *can* save the world, but your name doesn't have to be Patch. You too can break the rules of convention.

Thinking about the art of friendship is a fitting lead-in to talking about more specific art projects that can help you deal with illness and disability. As I think you know by now, the art in this book isn't for learning to do perfectly, nor in isolation from others. You might feel shy about asking personal questions of your doctor, but believe me, she'll have a hard time resisting you. It's an unusual joy for anyone who's devoting their lives to helping others to have a *two-way* relationship with a patient. But the chance for such a thing wouldn't have arisen in the first place, if not for the illness that brought you two together.

For the past ten years I've run what I call a "buddy program" between medical students and patients who have to stay in the hospital for long periods. This is the vital healing art of friendship at work. The crucial thing is that the students aren't part of the official health care team. They're more like extended family members giving the patient's wife or son or parent much-needed breaks from hospital visits. And they use art supplies and art-making to break the ice, so they have something specific to offer their patient buddy.

The students get a glimpse of the subjective side of illness, what philosophy professor Kay Toombs (1993), herself a person with multiple sclerosis, has called "illness as lived." They welcome the break from soaking up medical facts and figures. And the patients get the chance to develop a relationship with a caregiver that breaks through their conventional roles. Judging by its popularity, this buddy program is a welcome relief to many from long hours of boredom, or of anxiously wondering about their illness.

Surviving or Thriving

So what is health? Surely it's a lot more than just the absence of disease. If you define it as a balance among each person's physical, environmental, mental, emotional, social, and spiritual well-being, then it's quite possible to be in a state of overall good health, even if you have diabetes or cancer or heart disease. It just means that you've come to terms with your situation physically and emotionally; you've taught yourself about your illness and its treatment; you've taken charge of your treatment plan; you've built yourself a support system; you're still finding plenty of things to live for; and, most importantly, you've come to accept your situation, and perhaps make some sense out of why it's happened to you.

There's a lot written nowadays about *preventive medicine*. You may think this term doesn't apply to someone with an already established condition. But illness prevention (I prefer to call it health promotion) simply means taking charge of your situation and making every effort not to just maintain your current state of health, but actually to improve on it. Chronic incurable conditions can lessen in their severity and harmful effects, even if you can't get rid of them altogether.

Exercise: Your Personal Health Score

This exercise will help you look at your state of health, not your state of illness: what's *right*, not what's *wrong* with you. Some of the questions are taken from the book *Thriving* by Drs. Ivker and Zorensky (1997). Although it divides health up into body (physical and environmental), mind (mental and emotional), and spirit (social and spiritual), there's a lot of overlap between each of these different dimensions of health.

Give each question a score, either "0" if the answer is "never," "1" for "rarely," "2" if the answer is "sometimes," and "3" for "regularly."

Body (Physical and Environmental Health)

_____   1. Do you eat a healthy diet and drink a lot of fluids?

_____ 2. Do you take time to experience the pleasures of your five senses?

_____ 3. Are you free of dependencies on drugs or alcohol?

_____ 4. Do you nurture and appreciate your body?

_____ 5. Do you pursue any hobbies or physical activities for pleasure?

_____ 6. Do you feel energized by nature?

_____ 7. Do you sleep well and wake refreshed?

_____ 8. Do you challenge your body with physical goals?

_____ 9. Are you aware of life energy within you?

_____ 10. Have you benefited in any way from understanding your physical problems?

_____ TOTAL

Mind (Mental and Emotional Health)

_____ 1. Do you have specific goals in your life?

_____ 2. Can you concentrate easily?

_____ 3. Are you willing to take risks and learn from your mistakes?

_____ 4. Are you basically hopeful and good-humored?

_____ 5. Can you express painful feelings fully and appropriately?

_____ 6. Do you take time to relax and "let down"?

_____ 7. Do you use visualization or imagery to stimulate your imagination?

_____ 8. Do you enjoy any kind of art, either as performer or observer?

_____ 9. Can you adjust your feelings and attitudes as a result of painful experiences?

_____ 10. Do you experience feelings of excitement or exhilaration?

_____ TOTAL

Spirit (Social and Spiritual Health)

_____ 1. Do you commit a time and place in your life to spirituality and reflection?

_____ 2. Do you listen to your intuition and act on it?

_____   3. Are playfulness and humor important to you in your daily life?

_____   4. Do you make room in your life for children, animals, and growing things?

_____   5. Do you have close friends or intimates with whom you can talk freely?

_____   6. Do you use creative activities and art-making as an aid to deeper spirituality?

_____   7. Can you readily forgive yourself and others?

_____   8. Are you part of a community, and do you maintain long-term relationships?

_____   9. Are you grateful for the blessings in your life?

_____   10. Do you experience periods of peace of mind and tranquillity?

_____   TOTAL

_____   **Total Personal Health Score**

As a general guide, if you scored 75 or more, you're *thriving*. If you scored between 50 and 75, you're doing pretty well. If you scored between 25 and 50, it would be good for you to look at ways to enhance your overall health. If you scored less than 25, you're only just *surviving*! You could use a lot of help from family, friends, and caregivers, because you deserve a chance at better all-around health. I assure you there's a lot you can do to help yourself.

This questionnaire doesn't look much like the kind of questions I was taught to ask my patients when I was a medical student in 1960s London. But they stress this welcome trend in medicine toward self-help, in which caregivers and receivers, are seen as partners so people live the healthiest and happiest lives they can, whatever their circumstances.

Goal-Setting

This focus on healthy living—putting a high premium on eating and sleeping well, seeking healthy surroundings, spending time in nature, taking joy in your five senses, giving yourself regular physical and mental workouts, building community and taking time for friends and family, relaxing and contemplating the larger issues of life, enjoying games, hobbies, and culture, trusting your intuitive sense when making decisions—embraces some of the ways in which healing art is partnered with medical science today. In the next chapter you'll be taking a direct look at your natural creative abilities, and how you can use them for your overall well-being.

Although it's a good idea to set yourself goals, this is not about beating up on yourself for falling short. The American Cancer Society tells us that each time you give up cigarettes it's easier not to slip back the next time. I gave them up in my early thirties after fifteen years of smoking. It took me three attempts over the course of a year.

Exercise: *Your Health Issues*

Take another look at how you did in the above exercise. You probably had some areas where you'd like to have done a bit (or a lot) better. This is a follow-up exercise to help get you started with addressing some of these issues. Let your creativity fly in brainstorming possible directions and solutions. Put aside those "yes, buts . . ." that love to pop up and stop you in your tracks before you've gotten started. Affirm with yourself that for every possible problem in life, there is at least one elegant and fully accessible solution. Try saying it aloud: "For every possible problem, there's at least one elegant and fully accessible solution." Just remember that your resources are as much within you as external to you, and that the latter include human as well as material resources. But it's vital to set yourself deadlines as you determine to take action on what may well have become a long-term problem. So take up your workbook once more.

1. My health issues are primarily:

    a. Physical and/or environmental

    b. Mental and/or emotional

    c. Social and/or spiritual

    d. Equal parts of a and b

    e. Equal parts of a and c

    f. Equal parts of b and c

    g. Spread evenly between all three

2. I want to focus on these three issues:

3. These are some possible solutions or ways forward:

4. These are some resources available to me:

5. In the next week I will take the following steps to get me started:

6. Taking these steps will mean that I:

Look back over what you've written above, and add any further notes about what this will mean in terms of your current situation. It's important to be as precise as you can about these issues and what you plan to do about them. The last line of the list is especially important here. I stress again, though, that it's not about self-blame if you slip back. There's only one way to get started and that's by identifying the issues you want to work on, then committing to do so.

The Art of Healing

I recently interviewed an applicant for medical school: a woman of thirty-nine with one child a university sophomore and one a high school senior. She'd been a nurse for the previous ten years in a rural medical practice. Her husband had a secure position as an engineer in an expanding local company.

"Why on earth do you want to turn this fine life of yours upside down?" I asked her. "For four grueling years in medical school and three more in residency? Haven't you heard our profession's under the gun? That HMOs and insurance companies and big government are telling us what to do? That some good doctors out there can't even get jobs?"

"I don't care about that," she said. "I've learned about caring for people, and I know about life—misery and glory both. Now I want the knowledge, the science that medicine offers. Nursing can only take you so far. But I also know I've got something to offer that medicine badly needs. Healing is as important as curing."

This woman pinpointed for me health care's gathering momentum for a new marriage of science and art—a return to the *art* of healing. Medical science, for all its magnificent contributions, hasn't given us a healthy society. We are more than ready for the prescription this woman offered: the crucial ingredient of ancient healing art to complement modern medicine.

Story: Marie the Bald Beauty

Marie is a young woman of fourteen with bone cancer. She needed intensive therapy to stand a chance of being cured. Living as she did in a city some distance away, her visits to the hospital were protracted affairs. When I first knew her she had long, corn-blond hair that was her pride and joy. The anti-cancer drugs quickly had it falling out in clumps. She'd bought two expensive wigs, and would groom herself carefully before I or anyone else could come into her room. She would sit bewigged and cool through my examinations, saying only a couple of words.

Then one day she appeared in the clinic looking quite different. Not only was the wig gone, but she'd shaved off the last tatters of her hair. She presented herself to me with a proudly bald and gleaming scalp. Even more noticeably, she'd shed her inhibited manner along with her hair. She had once more become the cheerful and talkative self she'd been before. I quizzed her a bit about the new look. She answered right off that she'd just gotten fed up with those clinging wisps of hair, and with the wigs that did nothing for her anyway. She'd looked at her almost bald self in the mirror and come to the conclusion that she'd really lost none of her beauty. How right she was.

After that, until her hair finally grew back some six months later, she took great pride in her naked, shiny scalp. Sometimes she'd decorate it with face paint, which made for beautiful photographs. She took to helping the staff with the younger children in the clinic and on the ward. She introduced both them and the staff to the idea of not only face-painting but scalp-painting sessions. It got so everyone knew when beautiful bald Marie was in town.

Why Art?

It's hard to know what came first, Marie's new attitude or her new look. What *is* certain is that somewhere inside this shy teenager, who obviously felt isolated and angry both at her illness and its treatment, her artistic creativity reasserted itself. And along with it came a sense of control, a determination to make the best of her situation, and a commitment to help others do the same. Most of all, back came her sense of fun and joy in life once more.

Here are some very basic reasons for you to reclaim the artist within you:

- Art-making can help you function at your very best, even in the face of illness and adversity.

- It can reintroduce you to the delights of painting, music-making, dancing, and all manner of creative fun, just as if you were a carefree child again.

- It can help you express yourself emotionally, when words are hard to find.

- It can help you think more clearly when you have important decisions to make.

- It can build a community around you, for comfort and support.

- It can put you in touch with your very soul, the deep spirit within you that was there at the moment of your birth and will still be with you when you die.

Art and the Ancients

You might think these beneficial effects of art-making are a new thing. Quite the reverse: I'd go so far as to say that healing through art predates the practice of any other kind of health care that has been handed down to us. Some say it started in ancient Greece. It's true that the Greeks did make a strong link between creativity and health. During the poet Homer's time, about 700 B.C., music was well recognized for its pain-relieving properties. The hero Ulysses was healed of his wounds with chants as well as bandages. The mathematician Pythagoras made a daily practice of singing, because he thought it restored the proper balance among the four humors that Greek physicians believed made up the human condition. And at the Asclepian temples throughout Greece, music, theatre, and visual imagery through dreams were integral to the medical prescription.

But the Greeks didn't originate this medical practice. Art was a healing force way back in prehistory. As far as anyone can tell, human beings have always used pictures and stories, dances and chants, as healing rituals. The practice of art for healing in the ancient world made a universal link between the sick person and the forces of nature and divinity through the evocation of images. Psychologist Jeanne Achterberg, in her book *Woman as Healer* (1992), defines healing as "creativity, passion, and love, a lifelong journey toward wholeness, a recalling of things forgotten, an embracing of things feared, an opening of what is closed, a learning to trust life, a transcendence to an experience of the divine."

Those early healers—Siberian shamans, Asian mystics, priests of ancient Egypt, physicians of Greece and Rome—all used their power to restore this link with nature and divinity. They looked to dreams, images, and reverie as a way of healing. The creative arts have been preserved right up to the present in the traditions of indigenous peoples. In Africa, Australia, and Central and South America, dancing and drumming, chanting and meditation are combined in healing rituals to nourish both individual and community.

Lessons for Modern Medicine

Before languages evolved, humans most likely saw the universe through intuition and imagination rather than thought and logic. With language came the eventual flowering of science, alienating us from the natural world. There's evidence throughout the world that early healers helped tribal members interpret their own stories through drum and mask, dance and song, thereby purifying and revitalizing both individual and community. This persists today in all indigenous cultures, still the largest proportion of the world's population. Art is used *functionally,* not as decoration. Although many hours are spent creating an intricate sand mandala, for example, this is only in order to perfect its healing power. The shaman then at once sets about "using" the painting by walking on its surface and sprinkling meal on it. So the quality of the art, and of the artist, isn't the point at all. This is a vital thing for you to keep in mind as you start to make art your very own doctor.

Story: Europe's First Artist-Physician

One thousand years ago, Europe was emerging from the Dark Ages that had enveloped it after the fall of the Roman Empire. In a small town near Mainz in southern Germany, the noblewoman Mechtild gave birth to her tenth child. She called her Hildegard, and placed her in religious seclusion in a monastery as a tithe to the church. From early on, Hildegard was physically frail and susceptible to everything. Her only distinction was her gift for visions, but these were always accompanied by attacks of acute illness. During these episodes she found herself called on to tell about what she saw. Although at first she resisted, both out of humility and fear that she'd be considered in league with the devil, in the end she started to speak out.

From then on she produced many books propounding her visions, with help at first from a monk as recorder. These works took the form of original divine descriptions as well as stories with healing benefit for all who heard them. Soon she started to compose songs and poems, many of which survive to be heard today. She went on to blend natural science with medicine and music, becoming Europe's first medical artist-scientist. She always stressed art as much as science for achieving total health, and the themes of her books—on health, on spirituality, on nature—are all linked to her primary concern for planetary ecology. Most notable, despite struggles with her ailing health and political battles when she went on to found her own monastery, she lived to the ripe old age of eighty-one!

A Second Renaissance: The Body-Mind Connection

Hildegard's story is one of courage, creativity, tenacity, and faith. I hope it's especially heartening to you that her inspirations—her visions—and her subsequent productivity were richest when she was at her most physically frail. Unfortunately this renaissance of art and science in partnership was cut short by the Inquisition that swept through Europe in the thirteenth century, severing these ties for another five hundred years. Then along came Descartes the philosopher and Newton the mathematician to focus everyone's attention on science and technology as the only tools relevant to medicine, splitting mind and spirit totally from body, and setting the stage for the narrow scientific focus of twentieth-century medicine.

But belief in the unity of art and healing did persist down the years. Florence Nightingale, the "lady of the lamp" who founded modern nursing, reawakened this consciousness: "I shall never forget the rapture of fever patients over a bunch of bright coloured flowers," she said in 1859. "People say the effect is only on the mind. It is no such thing. The effect is on the body too." At the same time, scientist-philosopher Claude Bernard was advocating a balance between all parts of our bodies as being essential for total health. From his ideas, medical scientists before World War II began to sort out the effect of emotional stress on our many bodily functions, leading to today's detailed studies of the role of visualization and mental imagery in treating both mental and physical illness.

This body-mind connection has given rise to a new medical science that Dr. Robert Ader has termed psychoneuroimmunology (1981). It explores how the mind affects the body through immune, hormonal, and other systems. Lots of evidence now shows that your conscious and unconscious mind are linked to your unconscious physical processes, for good or ill. This is what forms the basis of the healing power of art-making, and so firmly links it once more to medical science.

Exercise: The Art of Relaxation

Here's an easy example for you to work on. Pick up a book from your shelf or bedside table. Make it an old favorite that's really gripped your imagination in an enjoyable way. Do you have one handy? If not, it would be good for you to gather around you a few such old favorites, especially if you're heading for a hospital stay. Children's classics are good companions for me: *Winnie the Pooh, Charlotte's Web,* or *The Just So Stories* are favorites. This is a great exercise to do just before you settle down to sleep at night, but it will work fine if you're in the habit of taking afternoon naps.

Now get yourself really comfy, either in bed or snuggled in a favorite armchair in a quiet spot. Make sure you're nice and warm, and that you're not going to be disturbed for half an hour or so. A little relaxing music will add to the cozy setting. Let the outside world drift away as you take a few deep breaths and settle in.

Open up your chosen book and look for a favorite passage. Or simply start right in at the beginning. Focus on the words in front of you. Use them to conjure up images of the scene, and the conversations between the characters. Let yourself "enter" the story, be part of its unfolding. If you find yourself getting sleepy, that's just fine. After all, that's what a bedtime story has meant for every child and every parent since storytelling began.

An excellent refinement of this exercise is of course to get your spouse or another family member or friend to sit on your bed and read the book to you while you snuggle under the bedclothes and drift off!

The State of Relaxation

This exercise can end whenever you choose, or whenever you wake up from the sleep (and its accompanying peaceful dreams) that it may well have induced. Was it a relaxing experience, diverting you from anything troubling in your current day-to-day life? I very much hope so. You can come back to this exercise as often as you like. It gets easier and ever more enjoyable with practice.

This state of relaxation is a physical thing, one in which your breathing slows, your blood pressure lowers, your muscles untense and slacken, your whole body "lets down." This is art—in this particular case, storytelling—at work for you. It's an art that creates images in your mind's eye, and this in turn releases natural substances in your brain—the equivalents of the drugs morphine, Valium, and many others that doctors normally prescribe to relieve pain and anxiety and so on. These natural chemicals, which their discoverer Dr. Candace Pert calls the "molecules of emotion," have been shown to have potent effects on the immune and hormonal systems throughout your body (1997). These systems in turn promote all your physical powers of healing.

So you see the integration of body, mind, and spirit has become a scientific reality. And art has been shown to play a central and holistic role in enhancing these mental, emotional, and spiritual effects on your physical wellness.

Healing Art:
What's the Evidence?

There's now ample evidence to support the ancient ways of using art-making in the service of human health. I'll review this in relation to each of the major art forms in later chapters. Here are just a few highlights.

The benefits of music therapy have been studied by modern health caregivers for at least half a century. Its benefits range from the newborn nursery, where it speeds growth and development in premature babies, to the end of life, where it is known to help relieve pain and anxiety. Music and sound have been used to relieve the effects of many other physical and mental disorders and disabilities that affect people throughout life. Music therapist Teresa Schroeder-Sheker's "prescriptive music" for dying persons has created a whole new art form, with its own training and licensure: that of playing harp music for those at the very end of life (1994).

The visual arts have healing effects in people with many health problems. Caregivers are recognizing the importance of aesthetically pleasing environments in speeding your recovery from illness. Architect Roger Ulrich showed some years back that a view of nature from your hospital bed gets you up and out of the hospital more quickly (1984). Paint, clay, and other materials have been used by patients of all kinds, helping them recover from injuries and strokes and supporting them in dealing with psychological and end-of-life issues. These art-making tools can become not only a joyful diversion from the hospital routine, but also a way for you to make sense of your circumstances, tell your stories, and move toward resolving the many problems and uncertainties with which illness and adversity may confront you. In her recent book, art therapist Cathy Malchiodi (1999) has brought all the evidence together.

Psychologist James Pennebaker is the leading researcher on the power of creative writing and journaling for bettering your health. He's shown that when you record stressful or traumatic events in your journal, both your mental and physical health improve (1997). It seems to work by strengthening your immunity. Your immune system may well be at the root of how all art-making helps you be healthier. It might be better called your healing system!

Then there's performance art. A great deal of research says that when you move and dance, laugh and play, it's as good as participating in sports and aerobics in improving both your emotional and physical health (Cousins 1989; Foster 1995). And performance art is a lot easier to do if you're stuck in bed or disabled in some way. Whether you're dancing or laughing, acting a part in a play or "playing the fool" as a clown, your mind is quite able to put aside your awareness of any emotional symptoms you may have, such as anxiety or grief, as well as any physical symptoms, like pain and physical weakness. Once more, your immune system seems to be at work.

Exercise: Creative Writing

Time for a little more art-making, this time in the form of your own words committed to paper. Take out your workbook once more. It would also be ideal to have some colored pencils available. You'll need some uninterrupted time; twenty minutes should do it. Try to ensure that no one will be needing you. Get away from the phone to a quiet, comfortable place. A little music is fine to provide a relaxing background, but it shouldn't be intrusive or distracting. Now take note: You need no previous experience. You won't get a grade, and no one is going to take a red pencil to what you write. No one will be scolding you with comments like, "Could do better." It isn't even necessary for anyone else to read what you write. It can be entirely between you and your inner self.

Become aware of your body. Notice your breathing. Follow your breath out and in. Keep bringing your mind back to your breathing and just follow it. Deepen it a little. Try to breathe with your diaphragm (your belly), opening up your lungs as fully as you can. Feel your body relaxing, unwinding. If you become distracted, gently draw your attention back to your breathing and your present situation. There's no hurry.

Now think of an occasion when you've been ill. Perhaps you're dealing with an illness or disability right now. Jot down in your journal as many details as you can: where you are or were, how old, who else is or was involved, what were or are your symptoms. List all the ways your illness has shown itself to you. Have you received any treatments? What has been helpful? And what definitely isn't or wasn't? Is there anything left of it now inside you? Can you describe that remaining part?

A lot of questions like these may come up in your mind as you get into it. Let them "appear," but try not to think too much. Keep your hand moving, writing from this imaginative place within you. It doesn't even have to make rational sense; just move it across the page. Trust your instincts. And always remember—no grades.

The Universe of Writers

As you write, notice this wonderful fact: You're a writer! It has nothing to with how good or how bad. You are actively contributing to the wonderful world of writing, of coauthorship with all the rest of us. This is a simple exercise in giving yourself *permission*, which is easier said than done, I grant you. You don't just have to decide it's worth your time to do something creative, you also have to get yourself to really relax into it. You've got to let time go for a while.

I hope that from what I've told you so far, you're convinced of the long tradition and the modern scientific evidence supporting art as health-promoting. I hope you'll start making a habit of prioritizing some creative time for yourself. If you're ill at the moment, this may be the most vital way you can spend your time. But it may take a lot of practice over quite a while to convince yourself permanently of this. It reminds me of a giant book that is right now being written all over the world by anyone who wants to contribute. Through a grant obtained by two Berlin artists, this book is traveling to many of the world's major cities, and being set up in squares and city parks. Passersby can write in it anything they choose, as a message to the world. When I caught up with it recently on vacation in Barcelona, seventy-three huge pages of words and drawings had already been filled by people from all over the globe, using many different languages. Yet the organizers said that their biggest problem had been convincing passersby that they had something to say to fellow human beings—or to themselves!

Exercise: Visualizing

Take this "sort of list" that you've just made of all the events and people concerned with your illness. Let your eye dwell on it. First use your outer eye—the one you use literally to read what's written on the page before you. Then after a few minutes bring your *inner eye*—that is, your imagination—into play. Let this imagination of yours make a composite picture of all these items on your list: a *snapshot.*

How do you *picture* your illness? As a cloud, or perhaps a rock? As a deep well, or a sharp dagger? Who's there in the picture you're making—are they friendly faces, or scary half-images of people? What about the treatment you've received? Does it have a calming, nurturing look and feel to it? Or does it look like something scary or chaotic in form? Now talk again on paper about the pictures you're seeing in your mind's eye. Describe them in as many ways as you can, filling in the details of the notes you've already made.

Take up your crayons and start to draw a picture of all that you've conjured up. What color and shape is it? How big? Does it have any other features? Is it just sitting there, or does it seem to be going somewhere? What about those other elements you wrote down, like the treatments that were helpful or definitely unhelpful. What did they look like? What about the other people involved? Where do all these different parts fit in your picture? What images and metaphors come up?

Look back over all you've written and drawn. You may well have covered a couple of pages or more of your workbook. Go back over it and add anything else that comes to you. Once you're done, put a date on your work, as well as a few words about where you are and what brought you there. This will serve to trigger your memory later.

Reflect for a moment on what you've created. This is visual and linguistic art. It's a creation, something conjured; these words and pictures you've made up are your very own works. Put them aside for now, but you can return and work on them at any time you choose. Like every other artist, you're only limited by your imagination, and there's no limit to that! I hope you're beginning to acknowledge to yourself that there's just no end to how much you can create.

Has this process of art-making changed anything in you? Notice if you feel any different. It may not at first be a conscious thing. But all the evidence tells us that the simple act of putting an experience of illness or adversity on paper, in words and images, is a healing thing. Perhaps it's because what you've created is in some way no longer a part of your inner chemistry. In putting distance between you and it, you've externalized it. This action, this process of art-making, has a weakening effect on any negative images or ideas that may have been lurking inside you. It loosens the grip that experience and memory may have on you. These are the sorts of memories that in time translate into physical illness, because negative or toxic experiences can cause permanent damage to your body's makeup. It's this sequence, which works first on your mind and then on your body, that art can reverse.

When and Where to Use Art

Have you wondered when, where, and how it's appropriate for you to put art-making to work for you? The simple answer is that this is your innate faculty for grappling with your past, present, and even future experience—positive or negative—and giving voice to it; so it's *always* appropriate for you to use art to express these experiences, in whatever way feels instinctively right. You don't have to be ill to benefit from creating art. Whatever your life situation, it can offer you comfort and companionship, diversion and excitement, insight and meaning. For myself, I can't imagine life without writing in my journal and scribbling poems, singing and dancing, making jokes and playing the fool with friends, family, and often patients. Every time I'm in my clinic, I relish the time I get to hang out in our art room drawing pictures, listening to music, and chatting in a nondoctor way to patients and families and volunteers.

But art's benefits are *especially* apparent at times when you're suffering emotional or physical pain, when you feel desperate or out of control. Illness and disability, within yourself or close family or friends, bring out these kinds of feelings. Many feel like they've become a child again in a world of adult alienation. That great bird of illness sweeps down on you, plucks you up, and drops you down in a strange country. This is the country of illness, full of new customs and language. Is it any wonder that children the world over use art to make sense of things new and frightening?

Perhaps most crucial of all, art-making can help you focus on enhancing your whole health all the time, rather than just reacting to and coping with any affliction or disability that comes along. It's a great thing to get in the habit of thinking of health as a *trinity*: that of your body, your mind, and your spirit. Even if your body seems to be giving way to some chronic disability, and even if there's no specific medical remedy to cure you and make you young again, never equate this with meaning you can't be healthy, in a holistic way.

Exercise: Your Last Breath

Imagine if you will that you're about to take your last breath on this earth. Conjure up the moment just before your heart's beat stills, your eyes close, and your lungs flutter down to their final resting place against your ribs. Is there any reason on earth or in heaven why this last breath can't be one of real *inspiration*? Why shouldn't you draw into yourself the divine creative spirit of the universe? Then you can become at last aware of the "holiness of the heart's affections, and the truth of the imagination" that John Keats spoke of. What after all *is* your whole health but harmony of body, mind, and spirit? Self-expression through art-making gives you the chance to find this harmony within you.

Simply imagine, for example, that you're confined to bed in an intensive care unit. Even in this situation it's likely you'll still be able to move some part of your body. Perhaps it's your eyes or the tips of your fingers. And you're likely to be able to do so in synchrony with the primal rhythm of your heart. There's a good chance you can follow this rhythm on visual display next to your bed! Now, how many ways can you think of to express yourself artistically in this last moment? How are you going to make a grand exit from here into the next world? It might be with a few loving or even joking words spoken to those gathered at your bedside. Or you could scribble them on a board in your lap if you can't speak because of the tube in your windpipe. How about something like: "I wouldn't change a thing, my dears!" Or "Nobody's going to tell me what to do no more!" And don't forget the use of sacred music, perhaps a harp, or whatever other instrument you especially like. Did you know that anyone can pluck the strings of a harp and make beautiful sounds? It's impossible for it to sound bad. You might want to die looking at beautiful pictures, or better yet, arrange for your bed to be by an open window, from which you can see and hear lovely sights and sounds of mother nature.

Nowadays everyone admitted to the hospital is encouraged to complete a form saying how they want things to be with them if it looks as if they're going to die. So envision for a few minutes how you would like to beautify your last few moments on this blessed planet of ours, for yourself and for those around you, when your time comes.

Choices in Art-Making

You may well be timid at first about expressing yourself artistically. Yet even if you are, you have the choice to be at first the "passive" recipient of art's healing balm and inspiration. There are as many forms of art-making as there are of self-expression. Beautiful images are or can be all around you. You need never be for long out of sight of the timeless grace and beauty of nature. You can provide for yourself a wealth and diversity of sound and music to strengthen and calm your mind, to give healing power to your body, and to plumb the depths of your divine soul.

Everyone will feel drawn at first to a particular way of appreciating and displaying their creativity through art-making. Later you may find yourself branching out into other ways of giving voice and expression to the artist within you. You may be wondering if one art form or activity is better for one type of illness or disability, and another for a different illness.

My own belief is that it's better to embrace art in all its many forms and facets. Don't get too *methodical* about it. Try all the exercises in this book at least *once*. And always remember that this whole process is not about judgment, about doing any form of artwork to get a grade. Whatever it is, you are choosing to do it. It's there to serve you—to inspire, uplift, relax, invigorate, calm, and harmonize you.

3

Resources: What Does It Take?

Creative minds will survive any amount of training.

—Anna Freud

Art-Making as Self-Help

So far I've introduced you to what creativity and art-making are all about, and I hope raised your interest in their crucial importance to you as a way of achieving the best health possible. You've done some preliminary exercises that I hope have planted the seed that you owe it to yourself to explore your creative instincts—if you don't want to rob yourself of your birthright!

I'm not offering you formal psychotherapy. But there are growing numbers of well-credentialed art, music, dance, drama, and poetry therapists, all blending the arts with the sciences of psychology, sociology, and anthropology to create a form of personal and collective therapy that Jung, the founder of analytic psychology, pioneered. Jung linked artistic images to subconscious meanings in the context of emotional and social illness. Art therapist Shaun McNiff calls art-making *soul medicine*: a medicine that allows the imagination to treat primarily your ailing spirit within you, and so *revitalize* you back from wherever you were failing (McNiff 1992).

Story: Hans the Survivor

Hans, a seventy-two-year-old German, is a retired army supplies storekeeper and a heart transplant survivor. He's also a survivor of the firebombing that swept through many German cities toward the end of World War II, and he's never forgotten it. "I remember a bomb exploding over our heads one time, and us kids running out of the building when the roof caught fire." His family emigrated to the U.S. shortly after the war. He reckons he can deal with anything life throws at him after those wartime experiences. But he also knows how close to death he's come since. "Before I got my transplant," he recalls, "I had one foot in the grave. And there's no guarantee my new heart'll last that long. They're in short supply too—there's always a waiting list a mile long. I don't know how they decide who gets the next one. Someone's got to die for us all to live."

He has to make frequent trips to the hospital for checkups, along with many other transplant recipients who are on the same life-long drugs to dampen their natural immunity and so prevent rejection of their donated hearts. "I've always been a sociable guy, and I soon got to know a lot of the people coming to the same clinic. So I organized a regular get-together. We'd sit around the waiting room after we'd had our checkups—two or three of us at first, but nowadays it can be as many as ten.

"At first we'd just talk about our illnesses and surgeries. Compare notes about the drugs we were on and the tests and all. But then we got into talking about our families and where we'd come from, old memories from our childhoods, things like that. With the stories I've heard in the last year since I started this I could have written half a dozen books." I suggested to him that maybe that's exactly what he should do: Write them down. In no time he'd have a book to show for this impromptu "support group" of storytellers he's created.

Your Repertoire of Resources

Hans and his fellow sufferers learned instinctively how the arts of group storytelling and mutual support can serve as informal psychotherapy. Their spontaneous initiative had the effect of *restoring by restorying* their spirits and minds wherever they were failing. It seems likely they went a long way toward re-creating healthier bodies too.

I want to take you on a journey of rediscovery of your own quite boundless ingenuity, imagination, and inventiveness. This journey will expand your ability to interact creatively, *artfully,* with your environment, with other people, and with yourself. In the process I hope you'll reclaim for yourself an even richer and healthier way of life. If you're at a place where illness or disability is putting limitations on you, this book has been designed very much with you in mind. The same applies if a family member or close friend is similarly affected, because they're looking to you for help and support.

Let's see exactly what it takes to put art-making and creative expression back into your life on a regular basis. What are the tools you'll need? Where do you come by them? Are they readily accessible or elusive? Will they cost a lot or be cost-effective? Can you really do this? How exactly? What kind of space will you need? Perhaps the biggest and most often asked question is, how much time will it take?

The repertoire of resources you'll need for making art includes things both *intrinsic* to you, the elements of your own creativity, and *extrinsic,* which includes not only materials but other people too. I'll try to show you how accessible these things are, and how you can make the best use of them, both as a source of personal support and in building partnerships with others. The kind of art-making I'm offering is not something you'll do a great deal of on your own. Partnering with others is an essential part of this process.

You have five resources available to you: intrinsic; environmental; other people; materials; time.

Resource #1: Your Intrinsic Qualities

By intrinsic I mean those resources that already reside within you. It turns out that these are the most vital of all. Without them, any amount of external resource won't move you forward very much. In many people, though, they've been neglected or suppressed. These are some of those qualities within you that I want you to give thought to, so you can value them and allow them back into your life:

- Your imaginative genius

- Your childlike curiosity

- Your artistic appreciation

- Your energy and passionate nature

- Your self-regard and self-pride

- Your autonomy and self-sufficiency

- Your love of nature and the earth

- Your vulnerability *and* your boldness

- Your gregarious nature

and most of all . . .

- Your instinct for making things up

This list may seem too simplistic for you to give much consideration to, because these innate qualities are the very ones you may have discounted. Yet each one is vital. Your imagination is alive and well every time you let your mind conjure up what the coming day may bring you. Your curiosity is piqued whenever you half-hear a conversation nearby and find yourself wondering about the speakers and wanting to fill in the details. Your artistic appreciation is awoken each time you look out of the window and take joy in the simple beauty of the sun shining on trees and flowers. And can you remember the last time you got all fired up about something? Perhaps it was a vacation you were planning or a surprise gift. Well, that was your energy and passionate nature at play. Your precious instinct for making things up comes into action all the time—whenever you compose a birthday or holiday greeting, write a thank-you note or letter to a friend, hum a little nonsense tune, put a plant in a pot, or make a meal from scratch.

The best way to get in touch with these intrinsic resources is by means of a couple of exercises.

✎ *Exercise: Letting Your Imagination Fly*

Here's an exercise in letting your imagination rip. It's adapted from one that four friends of mine made up and use a lot, as do I. They had each been deeply affected by family illness, which inspired them to write the book *The Healing "I"* (Block et al 1992), which has to do with what they call "self-help writing."

Take out your workbook and a pen or pencil. In answering the following simple questions, it's important that you write the first thing that comes into your head. Don't get intellectual on yourself. But it will add to the value of the exercise if you add a few specifics to your answers. For example, in answering question 9, rather than leaving it at simply "oak tree," try "a 100-year-old oak shedding fall leaves"—something with a bit more color and substance.

1. If I were a bird I'd be a _____ .

2. The one quality that best describes me is _____ .

3. If I were a city I'd be _____

4. If I were a car I'd be a _____ .

5. One thing I treasure in my life is _____ .

6. If I were a song I'd be _____ .

7. If I were a flower I'd be a _____ .

8. If I could have anything in the world right now it would be

   _____ .

9. If I were a tree I'd be a _____ .

10. One thing I could easily let go of is _____ .

11. If I were a smell I'd be _____ .

12. If I came back in another life it would be as _____ .

Did you manage to write down something without thinking too much about it? And did you write more than one-word answers, adding a little description about yourself as a car or a smell or a city or a bird?

To get the most out of becoming an artist once more, it's essential to respond like a child to the blank sheet of paper in front of you. We grown-ups tend to freeze at the sight of an empty space that we're supposed to be creative in or upon. That's not what serious-minded adults have been taught to do with their time—quite the contrary. Far from being scared by the blank page, though, any five-year-old will just go to it with pencils and crayons, starting right in with filling the space with the fruits of her imagination. The same goes with an empty physical space, like a playground or a yard: It's just made for dancing around and singing back to the birds in the trees!

So if you had a hard time loosening up in this exercise, you might want to take a big childlike breath and try it again. It's a fun exercise to do with a friend or partner too. Comparing notes always gets people laughing about the kinds of things they come up with. I did it with three medical student friends recently, and in answer to question 4 we all saw ourselves as sports car convertibles, although our colors were different. We decided it must be not because we're especially sporty types, but because we're all rushing through life much too fast, collecting speeding tickets on every freeway by gobbling our meals on the run and so on. So compare your answers with a friend's, and see what metaphors for life your answers throw up for you both.

Here's another simple (silly if you like) exercise, this time using pictures rather than words. Remember the old saying, KISS: Keep It Simple, Silly.

Exercise: Doodling

Using your workbook again and a colored pen or crayon, start a doodle going on a clean page. Let it meander where it will. Now try to take your eyes off it, or close them if it's easier, and let your hand go on its wandering. Don't try to direct it. Try not to pause or take your hand off the page. Keep going for two or three minutes, as if you were on the phone and your mind was preoccupied with the conversation. Let your eyes roam around the room, or just daydream if they're closed. Keep your hand as light on the page as you can. Cradle your pen or crayon lightly between thumb and forefinger and let it caress the page. Notice that it gets easier to be less self-conscious and more free-flowing as you get into it.

Take a look now at what you've created: all these random directions and connections, these fascinating shapes and patterns. Some will be faintly recognizable as an object or animal or body part—or even a person. Make a list of any familiar or not so familiar things you see in the images you've produced. Stretch yourself a bit—even a fragment of a pine tree or a truck, a whale or a human face or foot counts. How many did you come up with?

Start another doodle on the opposite page. The same rules apply. Take your eye and mind away from it, relax, and feel the weaving and wriggling of your wrist and hand and fingers. Breathe deep and free. Enjoy roaming over the empty space, like running across a field as a child. Okay, take a look again. Compare your two works of art. See how different they are (although if you're like most of us you'll have subconsciously tried to fill most of the space on the page). Again, count up all the fragments of creatures and objects you find populating your doodle. How many repeats from the first time?

Awakening Your Childlike Awareness

So now give yourself credit once more for being a creative being, one who can make rich use of your imagination, and who can make novel things appear at the drop of a hat. Not at all a bad skill, so I'd like to award you with the honorary degree of *MSU—Makes Stuff Up*—to put after your name.

This natural genius lies inside every one of us. See how readily accessible it is to you, and what huge fun it is to play with, like a new friend in first grade. The Romans saw our creative genius as our guardian spirit or angel, always hovering protectively near. This is a much more helpful concept than the modern distortion that ascribes genius only to the Einsteins and Picassos of this world. We all have our share of it to tap into, a much bigger share than we ever dreamed of. And there's no better time to reclaim it than when you or a loved one is ill or disabled, at home or in the hospital.

So I hope these simple-silly creative acts—of playing with word-images of yourself and describing them, and of making doodles and taking an imaginative look at the end product—have reawakened your childlike awareness and interest in the process. I hope too they've kept you focused (for a few minutes, anyway) in the present moment, without a care for what happened yesterday or might happen tomorrow. This is called being *in the flow*, as I'll talk about in a few minutes.

This kind of activity is definitely not something most of us devote much time to during our busy days. After all, you put your *curious child* to bed a long time ago, tidied her away in some dusty closet of your memories, like the toys you lifted for the last time off the nursery floor. But perhaps as you try these easy exercises and reflect on them, you'll find that creative child reasserting herself once more. Children faced with illness or adversity resort instinctively to art-making—writing, painting, making shapes and songs, playing with all manner of toys—to make sense of the strangeness, pain, and fear. This is a powerful inborn response, and there's good reason why it's built into us. It serves as protector and healer in times of crisis. What a pity it gets neglected and discounted in almost everyone as we grow up.

We adults would do well to take a few leaves out of children's books of art-making. Most children's hospitals have child life workers associated with them. Their training as health professionals teaches them to help children make sense of their illness, to understand and prepare for their operation or other treatment. They even help children prepare for death if they have an incurable condition. They always work with artistic expression, because it serves a profound purpose when words and concrete explanations are too hard to find, or too scary to hear. But the system hasn't seen fit to provide "adult life" workers offering similarly needed services to grown-ups. This is what artists at the bedside or in the clinic do.

Reflect back on the few minutes you spent on those last mindless exercises, playing those games if you will. Do you notice something else—that, while you were in the process of creating, your mind was not on the troubles or problems you may be dealing with in your life? If you have physical symptoms, perhaps you were able to distance yourself from those too. So take credit for taking charge of your health, and for deliberately distracting yourself from these problems and complaints, even if only for a few minutes. Give yourself a big pat on the back for the control you exerted over your situation and your environment. This kind of "escape," as it's often called, is a healthy thing. It has nothing to do with the kind of escape the drug addict or alcoholic engages in. It's the gift of art, lifting you out of the humdrum or perhaps painful and scary reality of your current life circumstances. It creates within you a new reality; actually, you create it entirely yourself.

Flow

The feeling of being engaged in art-making, what psychologist Mihaly Csikszentmihalyi (1990) calls being in a state of *flow*, is just like the practice of meditation. Meditation is mostly thought of as requiring dedicated training, perhaps in a Zen monastery, with regular sessions of sitting in a strict posture saying a silent mantra over and over. But try substituting the word *mindfulness,* or the phrase "being absorbed in the present moment." This is something you'll have caught yourself doing naturally from time to time. You can learn to do much more of it with a little practice. Art-making is a great lead-in to this blissful state of relaxation and present-time awareness. A New Yorker cartoon showed two Zen monks sitting cross-legged and side by side. The younger one is looking questioningly at the older one, who is saying to him: "Nothing happens next. This is it."

Dr. Jon Kabat-Zinn, who teaches *mindfulness meditation* at the University of Massachusetts, helps patients with all manner of ailments tune down their stress and anxiety levels by means of this acquired skill, and consequently boost their physical health. He sees this state of mindfulness as any activity—not just sitting still but walking, eating a nut, cleaning the stove, whatever—that achieves complete attention on the task at hand.

In his book *Wherever You Go, There You Are* (1994, p. 205) he speaks of cleaning his stove "with the help of Bobby McFerrin (on tape), the scrubber, the baking soda and the sponge, with guest appearances by hot water and a string of present moments." Cleaning has become dancing, the rhythms of the body merging, sounds unfolding with motion, modulations in finger pressure on the scrubber as required . . . "all rising and falling in awareness with the music. One big dance of presence, a celebration of now."

Seems like a pretty creative cleaning session to me. So here's an exercise that combines a couple of those in Dr. Kabat-Zinn's book.

Exercise: Slowing Down and Minding

You won't need any equipment for this. It's simply an exercise in being fully aware, or *mindful,* of your surroundings and of the present moment. This is the precious gift of creating. It brings us into awareness of what is ultimately the only thing we have: the present moment.

If you are able, take a trip outside. Walk around a little. If you aren't up to moving around too much, or you're stuck in bed, then your immediate environment is just fine. Take a look at what you see around you, above you, beneath your feet, even beneath your chair or bed. If you have a limited range of vision you can just recall in your mind's eye what's there, what makes up the totality of your environment. Take note, *without any thought or judgment*. Just notice—mindfully. Experience the feel of these things, a sustained feeling. How much of visual interest is there in your surroundings? Take stock. What do you hear? How many different sounds? Can you smell anything? Let your mind rest for a few minutes. Just be here with your surroundings, breathing them out and in. Let things slow right down, and rest in the present. See all these inanimate objects: stool, basin, curtain, clothes. If you're outside, take in the sky, ground, trees, buildings, flowers, and pathways as your very own peaceful companions. Enjoy them without hurry, without judgment, without any agenda. This is your environment, your presence, your life at this moment. It's the only moment you have. Breathe it in and enjoy.

Resource #2: Your Personal Environment

When you're ready, leave these few moments of contemplation and come back to the passage of time, and of your life. I hope you've enjoyed this spell of *time off*. Perhaps you've been able in this short period to appreciate how restful this slowing down and noticing is. It's in this place that your creativity and art-making will flourish once more. This is the world of the meditator, of the artist, and of the child. It's a place you can return to just as often as you like. And in this state you'll be alert and ready to respond creatively and flexibly to everything that happens.

Which brings us to your second resource: that of the environment that you create around you. The ancient Chinese called it *feng shui*. They used this term to define the art of creating an environment that balances you and optimizes your energy (Simons 1996). At its heart is your inner and outer harmony, keeping you in balance with your surroundings at all times, so that you can benefit fully from the *chi*, the healing energy of the universe that is accessible at all times to every one of us.

Story: Carl's Cell

I have a friend I'll call Carl. He's a psychologist, and he had to undergo a bone marrow transplant, a lifesaving procedure most often used for people with advanced cancer. Because of the high doses of chemotherapy and radiation he needed to his whole body, he was vulnerable to all kinds of infections and was confined for several weeks to a small isolation room, with very restricted space for moving about. The size of the space gave him limited opportunity to make it into a temporary home-away-from-home. But he started visiting his little "cell" a couple of weeks before he was due to be admitted, bringing in boxes of stuff that would remind him of home. By the time he was ready to move in, he and his wife had decorated every bit of available wall space with pictures and photos. He also brought his own stereo system and a set of CDs for all moods and occasions, his own chair, a small desk and computer, and even some bedding from home. Once he became aware of the view, which was of another large gray building less than ten feet away, he got some help rigging up curtains over the window. He arranged a system of signs on the door to say when it was fine for staff and visitors to come in, and when he was having private time and could only be visited in dire emergency.

Exercising Your Control

We often forget that we do have control over our environment. Sometimes it doesn't feel like it, especially if you have to spend time in the hospital. Actually, though, you can to a large extent set things up just the way you want them. This is especially important when circumstances seem to be taking away your control over things. If you do have to do hospital time, don't be deterred by feeling you'll be branded as a *difficult patient*. This is not a prison, even if it sometimes feels like it. You have rights! You are in charge of your life, even here. Just quietly but firmly insist on how you want things around you to be set up.

The modern Spanish painter Joan Miró lived to be one hundred years old. When he was almost destitute in Paris, still struggling at the age of fifty-five, and working in a cubicle so tiny he could hardly squeeze himself in, he said: "My dream . . . is to have a very large studio . . . so I can have lots of space, lots of canvases, because the more I work the more I want to work" (1938, p. 6). And that is exactly what he had by the time his life ended: a great big studio on the Mediterranean island of Majorca, just the way he'd dreamed it.

Everyone who aspires to being an artist needs to create their own environment for themselves. It doesn't have to be large or luxurious though. It doesn't have to be a whole room. It can almost be symbolic; that is, it can be a corner of your hospital room, say, that you've taken particular responsibility for, and in which you've collected all your icons and objects of special meaning to you. But it must be a place that's *yours*, that you have chosen and arranged and decorated. It should contain objects that are yours alone and have special meaning for you. Some call this a sacred space. The crucial thing is to see it as significant to you. Enter it as though you were crossing a threshold. You might want to use it as a place to be quiet, or to say a prayer, or to retreat to when you're sad or frightened. It might be a place to go to play, and to capture moments of happiness and success, or all of the above. Most of all, you might like to use it as a place for making healing art.

So now we'll do an exercise that will help you to create this special environment.

Exercise: Your Own Retreat

Pick a time when you're not going to be disturbed. Make yourself comfortable. Slow your mind down with a few deep "belly" breaths (breathing with your diaphragm). Just follow your breath out and in, until you begin to relax a little and let go of any physical or emotional tension. Close your eyes and be aware of each part of your body letting down, letting go. Let your facial features relax, then your shoulders and back, your pelvis and buttocks, your arms and legs, your hands and feet. Take a few minutes to do this.

Now imagine in your mind's eye a place of safety and sanctuary. This is your own retreat from the external world. Start to visualize where it might be and what it might look like. After you've read the list below, close your eyes and let your imagination go.

- Where is this place?

- How big do you want it to be? What are its dimensions and boundaries?

- What can you see when you are in this space?

- What objects do you want there with you? What especially personal things? Pictures? Photos? Your own bedding? Jewelry, or precious stones?

- What will you put on the walls? On the floor? A rug from home?

- Any furniture? A chair? A desk?

- What lighting?

- What can you hear? What do you want to hear? Music? What kind of music? Nature sounds? Rock and roll? Different sounds for different occasions? Or just blessed silence?

This process should take five or ten minutes. When you're fully done, let your eyes open, and bring yourself gradually back into the room. Take up your workbook and on a fresh page make a list of all these things. Title it "My Special Place" or something similar. Then sketch in your book a diagram of what it looks like. Yes, you're becoming an architect and interior designer too. Remember to let go of any judgment of how good your drawing is. It doesn't have to be to scale or even have straight lines. You may well want to use some of your crayons or colored pens to liven things up. Once you have your list and your diagram, make a date with yourself very soon to assemble everything and create your retreat. You may of course need some help with getting all these things together, especially if you're already confined to a hospital room or a nursing home.

Resource #3: Your Allies

Which leads us on to your third resource: that of other people, or allies. I discussed earlier the importance in today's health care scene of the doctor-patient partnership, and even friendship. I've also stressed that the kind of art-making I'm urging you to take up and practice is often best done with others rather than alone. There's good evidence that peer support groups are good for your total health, even adding years to your life span if you have a serious illness.

In our hospital's Arts in Medicine program, we lay great stress on working with patients and family members in groups. Making art together—whether it be scrapbooks or ceramic tiles, the squares of a quilt, a sing-along, or simply telling your stories—draws people together whatever their situation. In our society, with its stress on the individual in isolation from others, this renewed sense of connected-ness is at the heart of holistic health—the health of the collective as well as the individual. A support group gives you the chance to express yourself to others, to share your thoughts and feelings and confidences in a safe and nurturing environment. Making art of any kind offers an ideal framework for building this mutual support between you and others.

Allies and Rituals

You may find such allies among friends and family members, or, as is increasingly encouraged, among others in similar circum-stances to you, for example in a hospital setting. You may well find such support groups are available to you, but if not I urge you to cre-ate one for yourself and those around you, just like Hans the heart transplant survivor did. It may be just two of you to begin with, but that's fine.

It's good to establish a routine—a ritual, I prefer to call it—for meeting regularly, for example in a clinic waiting room or on a hospital ward if you're an inpatient. Meeting outdoors in a natural setting is especially appropriate if you can manage it. Rituals are often associated with religious forms and rites, but actually all of us perform rituals throughout our lives. Just reflect on your routine of preparing yourself for each day, of family mealtimes, of ending each day. These are all rituals, and they offer comfort from their very repetition. Reflect on how you like to maintain a particular order to the way you do things, as a way of grounding yourself, reassuring you that in this ever-changing world, some things stay the same.

Exercise: Time-Sharing

This is a brief exercise in ritual that I find useful whenever a few people, friends or allies or simply "fellow sufferers," gather together to share some time. It creates a sense of marking the time and place that you've set aside to be together. You can call it "checking in." It honors the process whereby people of all ages and backgrounds can learn to exchange simple but effective support and help.

Each of those gathered gets to spend two or three minutes introducing themselves and speaking spontaneously from an authentic place within them. This is not meant as conversation, nor as a time for comment or discussion. The others in the group should not prepare what they have to say while waiting for their turn to come. Rather, as listeners, they should pay full attention to each speaker in turn. Equal time-sharing is important, even if it feels a bit artificial at first. And this time-sharing should be accepted by everyone as confidential, which means that no one should bring up later what is said within the group. This creates the essential safety that any ritual activity strives for.

The vital thing in this exercise is that each of you *puts out* into the attentive silence your unique voice. You may want to reflect aloud on the current state of your life and health, or on what has been significant to you since you last came together. You may want to express some strong feelings, good or bad, in the safety of the group. You may even want to make commitments out loud to changes you're going to make in your life.

Your Internal Critic

When you try this exercise with a group or with just one other person, making it a habit of your coming together each time, you'll quickly experience the delight of this simple gift of sharing time. Like the place you created for yourself in the earlier exercise in this chapter, this ritual time together has about it a sacred quality that has nothing to do with any particular religious form or practice. It serves as an excellent prelude to a gathering for art-making, whatever your circumstances. In the sense that you gain a heightened awareness of the present moment together, it's similar in its effects to the ritual of meditation.

Another way in which alliance-building can be helpful is in overcoming your *internal critic*. This is an essential preliminary to all your creative activity, because it's the greatest bugaboo of all to letting your creativity flower. This critic is asserting itself any time you feel shy or self-conscious, or whenever you start to compare yourself with others and feel yourself falling short.

Self-doubt and self-denial have their origins very early in life. From toddlerhood you were in all likelihood stopped short of realizing your full potential by the wealth of judging and nay-saying and criticizing you received. I can say with some confidence that this happened to you, because it's happened to just about everyone who is now grown up, with a few stellar exceptions. It's the way our parents, and their parents before them, were taught to raise their young. It's only in the last few years that teachers and psychologists have begun to understand the importance of constant praise and encouragement in bringing up children. So this "negative" way of behaving was a powerfully reinforced lesson that we all learned well—that properly brought-up children don't brag about their accomplishments. You're supposed to accept any kind of praise with the greatest modesty, best of all deflecting it onto someone else as though you didn't deserve it.

The trouble is that by falling over backwards to avoid taking pride in yourself you end up suppressing your best most natural creative energies. You can't see yourself any longer as the hugely resourceful and imaginative being you really are. Do you think Miró or Mozart or Martha Graham or Lucille Clifton would have gotten any creative work done if they'd been forever plagued by modesty and self-doubt about whether they were any good or not each time they began composing pictures or music or dances or poems? And remember that when each of them started out, no one saw the genius in their work—except, I dare say, the artists themselves.

Exercise: *Taking Pride*

You'll only need one other person for this. It's an exercise in taking full pride in yourself, with a lot of help from your partner. The partner's task is to keep you on track with accepting some long-overdue compliments. You'll take turns of five minutes or so, starting lightly and working up to bigger things. Everyone knows their true talents, even if they don't acknowledge them to themselves, let alone take public pride in them. But some of you have never had your creativity acknowledged even as children, and you may well be quite unaware of your capabilities.

It's crucial that the listener—the praiser—pay constant and supportive attention all the time, urging the other on to shed their feelings of discomfort at receiving praise, praise that may even feel like mockery at first. Here are some suggestions to get you started.

Have a box of tissues handy, because you may find tears coming up. Settle yourselves as close together as feels comfy. Look right at your companion and make good eye contact. Whoever's turn it is to be in the supporting role starts by telling the one in the receiving role how creative you know her to be, that both of you really know this is so, even if she's never really acknowledged it to herself or to anyone else. Try at all costs to keep any trace of irony or mockery out of your voice, keeping your words and expression light but convincing. Levity with sincerity is the mix you're after.

Then step it up a bit, letting her know some things about her that you've always admired, and that you wish you'd gotten around to telling her sooner. Let her know how well she thinks about things, how imaginative she is, how courageous she is in trying to help herself and others around her. This exercise is about helping your friend get at her feelings of discomfort first, so her true pride can then surface. Keep going for about five minutes.

Then switch over and do the same thing in reverse. Expect to feel awkward at first. This is another ritual you're creating, and it may feel contrived. Accept the discomfort and push through it. Now that you're on the receiving end of all this praise, notice any memories that come up from earlier years as you get into it. Perhaps you'll recall times when you were discouraged or criticized. You may find a lot of emotion surfacing too: embarrassment, sadness, or anger at the way you were treated. Don't push it down, let it out (hence the tissues). Such feelings show you you're in touch with your authentic emotional self, perhaps long suppressed.

Okay, now you can both relax and bask in this renewed recognition of how *good* you are: how talented, flexible, smart, and creative. Stay together for a few more minutes, sharing together the feelings that have come up. They may be quite strong and quite negative feelings. Just let them be. Resolve to return to this ritual regularly whenever self-doubt and uncertainty are getting in the way of your being the artist you were born to be. This is an ideal start to a session of producing art together. I can promise you that your creative work will benefit from finally acknowledging your true ability—your genius.

Resource #4: Your Materials and Tools

Now we come to your fourth resource: materials. You'll become acquainted with the use of different art materials and tools during subsequent chapters, so I'm not going to give you too many details here.

It's helpful to divide the expressive arts into four major categories: visual, musical, performance, and language arts. Each one includes many different art forms, and they're often combined, as you'll see. *Visual* includes not just painting but clay-making and all other forms of sculpture, working with fabrics, origami (the traditional Japanese art of ornamental paper-cutting), making collages and jewelry, quilting, and so on. *Musical* includes both the use of musical instruments and also your voice for singing and sounding or chanting. Your voice is the most portable of all musical instruments! *Performance art* is any form of dance and movement, drama and mime, playing and clowning, so this covers a very broad spectrum of art forms. *Language art* is anything to do with writing, journaling, poetry, and storytelling, again a huge diversity of art-making.

It's a lot of fun to gather together a little collection of materials that will help you feel like an artist once more; these are just the sorts of things you might pick out for an eight-year-old child as a birthday present. It's also fun to do this with another person. If you're in the hospital, or preparing to go into the hospital, these are some of the items you might want to take along or have a family member or friend bring to you. Many people feel inclined toward one *medium* rather than another. You may want to start simply with the language arts or the visual arts, say, but I'll urge you repeatedly not to limit yourself to one form of artistic self-expression.

Exercise: Childhood Memories

This is an easy exercise to help you recall the creative times in your life and what came most naturally to you. Its purpose is to give you some guidance in where to start this process. How do you set out all over again on this journey of reclaiming on a daily basis the child-artist inside you?

Think back to the artistic things you liked to do as a child less than ten years old. Be as specific in your recall as you can. You may want to remember the art room at your summer camp or rainy vacation days at home. See if you can recollect crayoning or painting, writing in your journal or making up a poem. What about papier-mâché models or word games? You may have especially liked dressing up, even singing in a choir or performing in a Christmas play.

Use these memories as triggers to the materials you can surround yourself with. You may want to get yourself an elegant personal journal, in addition to the workbook you've been using up until now, in which to collect and tell stories with a companion or group. You might add a volume of favorite poetry to read from, either to yourself or with others. How about buying yourself, in addition to your box of crayons, some water paints and a few brushes, together with an artist's sketchbook? A tray of Sculpey modeling clay is a colorful and easy material to work with. How about collecting up all those magazines that accumulate in everyone's house and can be dusted off for collage-making?

These are all things you'll want to keep in the place you've set aside for your artistic endeavors. Chances are you can find a canvas tote bag from a workshop you or someone else was at. If not, they're very inexpensive in grocery stores. This is perfect for carrying your supplies around with you. We'll come back to material resources in later chapters, as specific art-making projects come up.

Resource #5: Time

Now we come to the last but not the least: *time*, a precious and undervalued resource. People who are ill become especially aware of it, in both a negative and a positive sense. On the one hand, if you have a serious illness you may have fears that time is running out, that you're not going to get better, that you won't ever be able to accomplish in your life all the things you once envisioned. On the other hand, illness is God's way of slowing you down. Becoming ill or spending time in the hospital does force you to put aside your busy schedule and all those lists and plans that you continuously make when your life is going along in its normal helter-skelter way.

The indigenous peoples of our world see time differently from those of us in Western civilization. We wear time on our arm, set our alarms to wake us at the same time every day, eat our meals at set times. We schedule appointments, meetings, and other activities in our day-planners weeks, months, even years ahead. This is quite foreign to the native American, indigenous African, or aboriginal Australian. To them time is universal, everlasting, sacred. You can best become aware of this in yourself when you use phrases like "I had the best time last night" or "This must be a hard time for you." Such a concept of time has no beginning, no set duration, and no end.

Re-Creating Yourself

The waking time left over from that spent on the essentials of daily life, and as your productive work time, is usually called leisure time. It accounts for about a quarter of your day. Oddly enough, this unstructured or free time is hard for many people to deal with, given the rules and regulations by which we've been taught to live our lives. Another often-used word for this is *recreational* time. The name implies that you should use this time for re-creating yourself and your life. But the huge leisure industry that has grown up in the past fifty years has the set intention of taking away from you the troubling business of facing this issue. It's robbed you of the responsibility of coming up with ways in which you can and need to *re-create* yourself during every moment of your free time. The result is that you never have to delve deeply into the issue of how you *really* want to put your leisure time to its most creative and rewarding use.

It's this kind of unmeasured and unstructured time that Dr. Csikszentmihalyi has highlighted in his writing about *flow*. Flow is all about experiencing optimal human experience. This is the state of timeless being that the artist and the athlete, the meditator and the young child, are well acquainted with. It is the state, or process, of being totally involved with life at this moment in time. The passage of chronological time becomes essentially shut out from your consciousness. For example, flow will inevitably overtake you when you are striving to achieve a goal or overcome a challenge of which you are *just* capable, but only when you put your abilities at full stretch. This is what transforms meaningless or boring or desperate lives into ones of conscious *re-creative* delight. Paradoxically, flow experiences, while being ones of great absorption that cause awareness of your present self and situation to disappear, will always leave you with a feeling of greater self-esteem.

But you don't have to subject yourself to huge challenges all the time to find the joy and focus that goes with flow experiences. It's completely accessible to you, to everyone, in regular small doses just like medicine! Illness, with the slowing down of your life that it inevitably brings, is an ideal time to reacquaint yourself with this kind of time and experience. And art-making is the ideal tool for this purpose. What it takes first and foremost is the simple, although not easy, *decision* to give yourself this gift: to set aside sacred time each day for indulging yourself in being fully engaged, focused, and *present*. This is the process of re-creating yourself. Re-creating, reclaiming, this time for yourself is as vital as creating sacred space—perhaps even more so. It's like learning to knit or ride a bike. Once you start doing it regularly, then it just takes the practice that inevitably comes with frequent repetition.

Let me make one thing clear though. Although flow experiences may well leave you unaware of the passage of time, that doesn't mean you can't assign a set length of time to your re-creation activities. It's perfectly fine to set aside, for example, thirty minutes each morning and evening, then let things happen spontaneously and creatively within that set framework of time, with your artistic materials at hand.

Exercise: Flow Experiences

This exercise will help you identify everyday experiences of your past and present life that tend to induce these *flow feelings*. The first stage is to make a list in your workbook of all the activities you can think of that give you, or have given at any time, the kind of pleasure I've described above. To qualify they should have had the effect of making you more alert, focused, sociable, motivated, fulfilled, or happy. It doesn't matter if they represent moments of high achievement or just of silly fun and fooling about. Anything goes as long as it gives you this kind of feeling, in small or large doses. One friend I invited to do this exercise said immediately, "Oh you mean like stretching out full-length at the top of a grassy hill in the park and rolling over and over all the way to the bottom?" Yes, that's it exactly.

Give yourself some fifteen minutes of uninterrupted time for this. Here are possibilities to get you started that might fill the bill for you: cooking a meal; mending something that's broken; reading an exciting story; gardening of any kind; grooming your hair and nails; telling a good story to your neighbor; playing any outdoor sport; playing a board game or completing a jigsaw puzzle; sewing a dress; working on your car or bicycle; writing in your journal; putting together a new outfit; singing in the choir; making new friends; going for a drive; solving a dispute in the office; exploring a new vacation site; saying your prayers; watching a gripping movie; throwing a party; comforting someone who's hurting; learning a new dance; studying your favorite subject in school; hiking in the woods; sunbathing; playing with a pet; swimming in the ocean.

And so on—there's absolutely no limit to the possibilities. The crucial thing is to delve into your experience of life for long enough to come up with a list of at least twenty different activities that work for you. But always keep it simple. The next stage is to look over your list and order all these items in some kind of priority, so that you can get a fresh realization of what things really turn you on. You might even want to score each one on a scale of ten points, although you don't have to get into such detail. Just be sure you have at least half a dozen activities out of your life experience that are likely to give you a taste of flow. And of course they have to be accessible to you in your current life circumstances, even if they need to be modified somewhat.

Now take a look at your top ten. See if you can find some common links among them. How many are more physical than mental? Are most more left-brained than right-brained? Are the majority more outdoors than indoors? How do they break down in terms of being solitary activities, or ones with one other person, or with a crowd? Perhaps most significant: how many are almost confined to your past life as opposed to your present one? This will tell you a bit about those kind of pleasurable pursuits that you've let drop, or perhaps felt unable to do anymore because of lack of time or ability. In future chapters I'll show you many easy ways in which, using art-making in the broad sense of the term, you can nourish those parts of yourself that have gotten dusty from disuse.

4

Imaging and Imagining

The most important form of communication is visual.
Our dreams, visions, and drawings speak the truth to us.

—Bernie Siegel

Images in Our Lives

Visual images are part of our waking and our sleeping lives. Like it or not, we're surrounded, often bombarded, by them. They may assault us, get in our faces with their wish to tell us, or sell us, something they claim we can't afford to miss.

Our earliest forebears knew the powerful restorative effects of visions, and of making pictures—images or visual art—from them. They decorated their cave-homes with primitive shapes and symbols we can still marvel at, so many generations later. The simpler they were, the more arresting we find them. That's perhaps why our dreams, however transitory, are often larger than life. They capture our subconscious attention with the size and strength of the visions they lay before us.

Story: Painting Her Way to Health

Brenda was forty-two when she developed a rare condition called aplastic anemia. For no good reason her bone marrow, where blood cells are made, stopped pumping out its daily supply. The severe deficiency of red cells, white cells, and platelets that resulted brought on a whole array of symptoms: tiredness and weakness from the profound anemia, debilitating and dangerously high fevers from her lack of immune defenses, and ugly bruising and heavy vaginal bleeding from her lack of ability to clot her blood.

Worse than the specific symptoms themselves, Brenda told me, was the unspeakable strangeness of it all. Neither she nor her husband could begin to make sense of this invader that was suddenly devastating their well-ordered lives. "It was as though I'd gotten up one morning, gone out of my house, and found myself in a strange country where no one spoke the same language as me." That's how Brenda described the effect on her life as a successful realtor and mother of three teenagers of finding herself almost overnight unable to cook the family meal or keep the house picked up, let alone keep working or staying abreast of her normal stream of day-to-day activities.

She was perhaps no different in her experience from the multitude of others that life-limiting illness strikes with such sudden force. But even as her doctors described the seriousness of her plight, the limited choices of treatment open to her, and the none too great chances of recovery, Brenda found comfort in having at last some understanding of what was going on, in knowing what she was up against. She realized suddenly that she wasn't the only person in the world to be struck down with such inexplicable misfortune. She may have entered an alien country, but at least she was starting to grasp a little of the language, to find ways to make herself understood to her cast of caregivers.

She saw that, at least for the moment, she would have to let go of a lot of her life up until now—its fast-paced schedule and host of different responsibilities. "I just had to put myself in the hands of these others, not just of my family but of all kinds of total strangers. I'd been used to being in complete charge of my life. Now suddenly I couldn't control things anymore." It was then she started painting. She couldn't recall afterwards exactly when the notion took hold of her. "I think I just woke up one morning out of a dream of myself picture-making as a little girl of about six years old. That's certainly the age I'd been feeling recently in my real life—as though I'd just entered first grade, a new and very scared kid on the block. With no experience, no fellow-sufferers, no savvy.

"But once the first horrors of the bone marrow tests and the blood draws, the antibiotics and transfusions, had slowed down a bit—had become more of a kind of background rhythm to my days—I suddenly found I had a lot of time for myself. Time for relaxing a little bit, for reflecting and daydreaming some. I was still getting bouts of feeling pretty crazy, but at least it didn't look as though I was going to die tomorrow. And I knew I couldn't do much, if anything, about what was going to happen in the future. So I just started to think about making the best of my day."

She was spending her days either in the clinic or overnight at the hospital. She got into the habit of packing her overnight bag for each visit, complete with a sketchpad or some loose pieces of paper, paints, and brushes. They didn't take up much space, either in her bag or in the clinic waiting room. She didn't know anything about painting *technique*, and some contrary part of her—the defiant six-year-old perhaps—refused to learn much of anything about it. All she wanted to do was just make colors on paper, great splotches and swirls and nameless shapes. "It was comforting, sort of safe. I didn't have to explain it to anyone, I could just run away and hide with my paints and my paper. They were my friends. It was like I could tell them anything I was feeling and thinking. They didn't answer back, didn't give me bad news, didn't counsel me about what was best for me."

She made hundreds of these pictures, some brightly colored, some dark and somber. "None of them had titles, and you could see whatever you wanted to in them. I didn't need to interpret them. They were just like a child's paintings, which was exactly what I wanted them to be like. Somehow, feeling like a six-year-old again not only had its painful and scary side, but it was also kinda fun, once I got into it. Sometimes I'd feel guilty and worry about my husband, let alone the kids and my work at the office. But some part of me kept reasserting itself, telling me to just 'let go and let God.' Who'd have thought it?"

Letting Go and Letting God

Brenda is a great example of an adult coming to terms with illness through art. She was *led*, because no one suggested it to her, to pick up paints that had been laid down several decades before. She made absolutely no pretensions to talent or technique, had no particular ambition pushing her in that regard. She actively denied any striving to make her paintings *better*. That was definitely not the point, any more than entering into extensive psychoanalysis to figure out what they meant.

This is the very beauty of art for healing purposes. When you let go of the need to achieve, or even to understand at an intellectual level, you give your ego a rest, and so throw yourself slap back into your very young childhood again. It's a thrilling ride, believe me. You'll be back in the time before you were first socialized to this need to succeed, to make a competition out of every leisure activity. You'll be back in the time before you needed to analyze and explain everything for the sake of a higher grade. This is true *re-creating through recreating*—coming very close to the original genius we were born with, a deeply spiritual place. What Brenda was doing in making her pictures was something akin to meditating, or praying. It was just like being *in the flow*. Because you can think of this state of flow as your immersion once more in that underground river of awareness inside, where your soul lives. It's always there waiting for you, when you're ready to dive in.

The link between Brenda's illness and her turning to art is simple and inescapable. There she was, feeling like a child in all her impotence and helplessness, and then suddenly her instincts—she seems to have called it God—prompted her to turn all this to her advantage. I sometimes get to wondering why everyone doesn't do the same. Maybe Brenda did have more support in her endeavors than some, but she also had more *adult stuff* to let go of than many. The Yale University surgeon Bernie Siegel, in his book *Love, Medicine and Miracles* (1986), speaks of how he's always urged his cancer patients to draw images of their illness and its treatment, so they can get in touch with what they really believe about their situation, and what this authentic self knows is best for them to do about it. This is their own internal therapist at work on their behalf.

As far as I know, Brenda's never sought to explain or analyze her artwork, nor to demonstrate any pretensions to Jungian psychology, which is based on the harmonizing of conscious and unconscious. The process of making art spoke for itself. Just to watch her at it, sleeves rolled up, hands and often clothes daubed with splashes of paint, like a palette, was comforting even to a mere observer. It slowed you down, pushed your own external world gently away a pace or two. Meanwhile she was able to discover instinctively within herself what was best for her to do as she made sense of her situation. She truly took charge of her illness and her treatment.

Imagination and Your Health

There is growing scientific support for the beneficial effects of imagery on your health. Physicians and psychologists are coming to accept that the images of an ill person can communicate feelings and less obvious symptoms in ways the conscious mind can't begin to appreciate. A landmark book is *Getting Well Again* (1981) by the Simontons and James Creighton. Two later books—Achterberg and Lawlis' *Imagery and Disease* (1984) and Dienstfrey's *Where the Mind Meets the Body* (1991)—discuss the many positive effects on your immune system of creating visual images in your mind and on paper. It's this immune system that's your primary protector against both infections and the growth of cancer within your body. Biofeedback, a well-known technique psychologists use to train your mind to control your bodily processes, also relies on your innate capacity to visualize internal processes associated with thought, relaxation, and creativity.

How Visual Art-Making Is Used for Healing

I highlighted in chapter 2 some evidence for using the visual arts to help you when you're ill. First of all, it's clear you need to create *aesthetic* (artistically pleasing) surroundings for yourself, if they're not there already. Simple views of nature scenes can hasten your recovery, for example after an operation. Other studies have shown that the choice of art in your room is very important to your well-being. Using different types of art on your walls has a positive effect on your emotional health. Some images seem to have healing effects on everyone who spends time looking at them. Good examples are scenes of forests, waterfalls, oceans, and rainbows. The effect of other visual art depends more on individual preference, and this can in turn be affected not just by your personal tastes but also your life experiences. This is a subject that needs a lot more research, as hospitals and caregivers refine every aspect of the true meaning of healing.

Hospital and nursing home architects, designers, and administrators are increasingly working with artists to create buildings that are not only efficient but beautiful, restful, and harmonious too. Simple and pleasing signage for finding your way around has become an art form in its own right. This modern renaissance stems from a renewed interest in the ancient Chinese art of feng shui I mentioned in chapter 3. Feng shui explores the design, placement, and color of objects in your internal and external environment, so as to harmonize the universal healing energy, or chi, around you and within you.

All of this has to do with the passive enjoyment of visual art and its beneficial effects on the viewer. Actively engaging in the process of making art probably has even more powerful effects. Both adults and children with health problems ranging from AIDS and cancer, injuries and strokes, emotional and end-of-life issues have been shown to benefit significantly (Malchiodi 1999). The profession of art therapy has become well established since the 1950s, although there are still far too few art therapists in our general hospitals. All kinds of art materials and activities have been widely used in these settings. They include colored chalks and charcoal, pastels and paint of all kinds, clay for simple sculpting, quilt-making, the Japanese art of paper-cutting called origami, and collage-making.

Dr. Robert Coles (1993) has led the field in showing the value of art in health education. The arts and humanities are now widely taught to medical and other health care students, to foster a more humane and caring approach to the work of service. I've stressed already that this modern movement has its origins in the age-old customs of indigenous peoples. Our native American tribes have always used ceremonies of bodily decoration and sand paintings, as well as dance and chant, for their sacred healing powers. The relationship between body, mind, and spirit for total health is the basis of the healing rituals called *sings*, which include the traditional Navajo songs, poems, and creation of sand paintings. These ceremonies help sick persons visualize themselves as healthy and in harmony once more with the universe. The beauty and simplicity of consciously making your own visual images—your own art—is that you can do it in any way you want. You're in charge. No one is there to judge you. What a blessed thing, at a time when you're no longer in the driver's seat, to have something fun and fulfilling that you *can* take charge of.

Exercise: Choosing Your Art-Making Materials

This is an exercise in getting acquainted with the visual art materials you'll need, in a way that will take some of the fear of the unknown out of it. If you've already made up your mind to equip yourself with some of these tools, you may have felt intimidated by the very abundance of everything on display in your local art supply store. But it's essential that this be a fun experience. I don't want you to get turned off from art-making when you've only just begun.

So, if you're able, gather up an interested friend and plan a trip to your local art supplies store. Actually, you can immediately remove a lot of the threat of this by going to one of the larger drug stores or a school supply or toy store. Office supply and copying centers also have a lot of the supplies you'll need. If you can't because of illness or disability make such a journey, this exercise will serve to help you create a list of things a friend or family member can pick up for you. Or you can use the many supply catalogues that are available today.

Don't feel like you have to get everything at once. It's not only cheaper but less overwhelming and more fun to accumulate things as you go along. It's a good idea, though, to make a preliminary list of what you think you'll need, based on your own inclinations and what you've read so far in this book. The first thing to do when you get to the store is take a good look around and see what's there. Pick everything up. See what it feels like and what its purpose is. What attracts you and feels pleasurable to handle? Even check out how it smells. On the other hand, what feels daunting or too foreign to you? Start making a list of questions and clarifications, to ask at the front counter if you're in an art supplies store. Don't be too shy to come up with simple-silly questions.

To start off, you'll need a box of crayons (Crayola makes a box of forty-eight three-inch ones); and a box of chalk or oil pastels (they come in twelve or twenty-four mostly); and/or some soft drawing pencils, which can also be colored. A set of highlighters in four or five different colors is also nice to have. Make sure you equip yourself with paper clips of assorted colors, as well as a stapler and erasers. You'll need a pair of scissors and some glue for pasting pictures on to cardboard or perhaps into your workbook or sketchbook. There are very convenient (and nonmessy) glue sticks for this purpose.

If you want to try your hand at painting early on, get either acrylic paint, which dries quickly and can be painted over, or tempera, which washes off most things easily. The store clerk can line you up with a few student-grade paintbrushes. You'll also need containers and rags or sponges, which you may be able to find lying around your house. For surfaces to work on, you'll find a choice of papers, and you can also work on cardboard, which accepts most of the above and is sturdier. You already have a workbook, and perhaps a separate journal, but you might want to have a sketchbook too. You should also get some multicolored Fimo clay or Sculpey, which is a plastic modeling clay you can fire in a toaster oven. It's fun and easy to work with, and great for keeping stiff fingers more mobile.

The next thing you need to do is start your collection of *found art objects*. This can be as big as your imagination lets it be, as long as you have a place to store the many items you collect and may want to display from time to time. I'm talking about interestingly colored, shaped, or textured pebbles, leaves, feathers, twigs, and bits of metal. Buttons, beads, shells, colored glass pieces and thread, and assorted foreign coins are also fun to collect. Absolutely anything goes that looks good, feels good in your hand, and attracts your imagination. Get into the habit of seeing the intrinsic beauty in these objects. Many people don't need coaxing to pick up these things on walks through the woods or on the beach. You'll be using them to weave into pictures, sculptures and jewelry you'll create along the way. You'll be adding them to magazine images that catch your eye, inspiring you to cut them out and save them. They're probably best kept in a pile in a separate shoe box.

Now you have the fun of gathering up all these things and putting them in order, making a home for each of them in your sacred space of art-making. Just to look at all these new friends each morning will quickly lift your mood and put you in tune with your imaginative artist-self.

Exercise: Imagination: What Does It Do for You?

This is a preliminary to the exercise that follows, which is about becoming aware of the endless river of images passing across your mental landscape.

Start with a blank sheet of your workbook or sketchbook, and with a crayon or chalk make two columns by drawing a line down the middle. You're going to list all your beliefs and all you've been taught about your imagination. Take a few big belly breaths to settle yourself and loosen up emotionally. Then start right in by writing down any phrases or short sentences that come to you about this one word: *imagination*. As you do this, assign each one to the left or the right column, according to whether they strike you as negative or positive ideas or statements. For example, under negative you might list such phrases as:

- "It's just your imagination."

- "Your imagination's running away with you."

- "You just imagined it."

Do you notice how each of these common expressions has a derogatory feel to it? They're really put-downs. Now, in the positive column, you might list statements you've heard somewhere like:

- "You're so imaginative."

- "Imagine you could have anything you wanted."

- "I wish I had your imagination."

Notice these are, on the other hand, words of praise. Got the idea? From just these few examples you'll see that this simple and seemingly harmless word arouses some very mixed reactions in people. Take five or ten minutes to complete your two lists. Dig back into your childhood memories a bit, to when you first heard the word imagination, from your early teachers perhaps. Then focus on more recent times when you've heard it or seen it written. Now take a look and see which of your two columns is longest; in other words, whether the word has a positive or negative connotation for you. If you score on the negative side, don't be surprised or discouraged— most people do. It seems we've been taught to devalue and even deride the use of imagination in our society.

Exercise: Capturing Your Images

Now you're going to start actually pinning down your images in your mind and learning how to put them into external form on paper. You'll need your crayons, colored chalks, or chalk pastels, and a fresh page of your workbook or sketchbook.

You're going to be making spontaneous and quick scribbles, or primitive drawings if you will, of whatever images you see before you as they flash by. Open the box and let two or three colors grab you. Try not to choose. Let them choose you. That way you're already starting to let your intuitive self take charge, and telling your thinking self to take a nap. You'll need to read the instructions for this exercise ahead of time, because you have to close your eyes while doing it.

With your colors in hand, or immediately handy, close your eyes and let the sequence of moving pictures start to appear. If you have trouble getting into it, a good trick is to take a firm stand against letting anything appear at all. As soon as you decide to maintain a blank screen, you'll like as not be bombarded by images of all kinds. If I say to you, "Whatever you do, don't imagine a baby pink elephant scampering through the undergrowth toward you," I defy you not to conjure up just such a picture of a dainty little elephant of that very color.

Focus your eyes very close in front of you, as though on the *canvas* of your inner eyelids. Hold this focus steadily. What do you see? It may seem completely dark at first, like the stage curtain of a theatre just after the auditorium lights go down and before the curtain goes up. Just stay with it and let the images come, right onto your personal stage or movie screen. Let them float or hurry by your *inner eye*. They may come in from the sides or appear along a kind of tunnel out of your head. Just note them and enjoy them, but don't think too much about them or judge them.

After a while, with a bit of practice and on a good day, you'll find these images pouring onto your screen. Notice their variety, and oftentimes their apparent meaninglessness. This is an art gallery of your own internal work. All these pictures are made up by you. As the pictures start to show up on your closed lids, start to work with your colors on the paper. Be ready to turn over the pages as you go along, but don't open your eyes. This way there'll be less interruption to the flow, and no censuring of what you're producing. Don't worry—

they may be unrecognizable to anyone else, but you'll know what you saw, and that's the fun of it. Don't get too caught up in capturing each image in detail on the paper—just a few lines will usually do. See if you can make about half a dozen pictures in five minutes or so.

A Picture a Day Keeps the Doctor Away

Okay: When you feel ready, take a few more breaths, finish up your last picture, and open up your eyes. See what you've got, and as you look over your art gallery, notice how easily the images come back to you. This is your imagination at your service. Notice too how restful this is. Like all the exercises in this book, it will get easier and easier with practice. This example is the simplest kind of playing with visual art. You can return to it as often as you like. Indeed, it's good to get into a regular habit—a daily ritual—of doing some unstructured, colorful image-making. Otherwise you'll slip back and start neglecting your new friend. This is what most of us do all our adult lives, and we lose the health benefits it can promote. Like eating an apple, creating a picture a day may well keep the doctor away. Wouldn't it be great if you got into the habit of spending ten minutes dabbling with colors and images at the start and end of each day? This isn't such a demand on you if you're laid up and have some time on your hands; it's a *date* to look forward to every day. Believe me, the healthful rewards of getting your internal pictures down in visible, external form are immeasurable.

Exercise: Image-Healing

Once you've got the hang of capturing some of the images that float onto your personal movie screen, you're ready for something a bit more structured. You're going to explore image-making for personal healing.

You'll need your sketchbook or workbook again, and wax crayons or chalks. Or you might like at this point to venture into paint. You'll find something joyful about dipping a soft brush into a little cup of water, and the extra freedom it gives you to splash some color around. So what if you get a bit spilled on your clothes? Just don't put on your Sunday best (or your best nightie) for this activity. And pick a time and place where you won't be disturbed for thirty minutes or so. If that's hard to set up, you may have to gently but firmly insist on it. It's fine for the moment to experiment on your own, although you'll soon find out what fun this activity can be with companions.

An ideal place and time is outside on a starry night at bedtime. You may have to wait a while for this starry night, and if you're "confined to bed on doctor's orders" then perhaps you can get someone to wheel you outside. The great thing about gazing up at the stars is that it's a marvelous practice for looking beyond what you can see immediately. First you focus *on* all those myriad stars, then you try to look *through* and *beyond* them.

Now it's time to breathe. Get yourself settled and quiet things down around you and within you. Loosen or untuck your clothing. Now try ten breaths, deeply in and out, lowering your diaphragm down deep into your abdomen with each in-breath, consciously letting the out-breath continue as long as it will. But don't work too hard; just relax into it. Now gently close your eyelids once more, and start to let the day that has just passed come into focus. But see it as a series of color images: each event, whether happy or sad, anxiety-provoking or comforting. And see in your mind's eye once more each person you've talked to, either to pass on some news or to chat idly with. Or it might be someone with whom you've had a disagreement or a fight.

When you're ready, open up your eyes and your paint box or box of crayons. Get your cup of water and dip your brushes in. Start putting some of these images onto the real-life canvas in front of you. Don't choose too consciously. Let one suggest itself to you, once more exercising your intuition. Try to keep yourself as far as you can in your nonthinking, nonjudging mode. Above all, don't worry about making things that are necessarily easy to identify. Play with the colors you have available to you. If you don't have a big assortment, you can put that right before next time.

This whole experience is an experiment in working with shapes and colors for their healing effects. You may not have thought for years about which colors you like best, or noticed how they blend together. Actually you do think about it, but mostly subconsciously, every time you get dressed and try to match your clothes up. But now you can just have fun with your mixing and matching. Try to match colors and shapes to the pictures of the day that are presented to you. You can make as many images as you have pages to paint on. It's an especially good idea to use several pages if you're the sort of person who tends to use up very little space—the economical sort. Go on, be extravagant and spread yourself out a bit.

Now compare your images. See what colors and shapes are pleasing and soothing to you, and that you can use to depict a pleasant image. Then notice which shapes and colors are harder and more confronting, to depict moments or people that disturbed or upset you during the day. You can crumple any one of them up and toss them in the trash as you make them. And you can keep back a few that appeal to you. Don't hesitate to rip pages out of your book if you want to, because there's more where that came from.

This exercise is the visual equivalent of keeping a journal. It helps you externalize anything left over from your day that you want to *take note of* as being of comfort or particular significance. You create images of matters that you need to resolve, so they don't keep you awake at night or pop up again first thing in the morning. This can have a profoundly relaxing and cleansing effect on your mental state. As you've learned, this can be crucial to your physical healing. You'll also be astonished at the hidden stories and meanings your pictures will present to you. These can be of enormous help in giving you insights, understanding, and help in decision-making—whatever your life situation.

Rituals of Color, Shape, and Texture: What Works Well?

Here are some of the activities using visual art that the artists in our Arts in Medicine program use. These have proved helpful to patients and their families of all ages. Painting on clothing—plain caps, visors, and T-shirts—is a favorite activity. Fabric paints cost about a dollar each at craft stores. You can stretch a plain T-shirt over a picture from a book and trace the outline before filling it in with your paints. Or, better still, you can just paint using your imagination, as you get more and more confident in its unlimited potential.

Our artists also encourage groups of patients, staff, and volunteers to make murals together. A mural doesn't have to be painted directly onto a wall, although that's ideal, assuming you're using paints that can be washed off. Several of you can quickly break down a giant piece of paper into manageable parts. Before you know it you'll have a communal art piece you can all take pride in. To be quite sure you don't get competitive or intimidated by each other's efforts, it's fun to rotate a painting at frequent intervals and work on each other's sections. This way of making art together is not only a lovely way to share some time, it's also the easiest and surest means to overcome the inevitable inhibitions that "nonartists" feel about making art after a long break from it (perhaps all your adult years).

For the last several years, patients, families, and staff have been decorating wall and ceiling tiles around our hospital. It's become almost a way of life for anyone who wants to do something collaborative, and there are a lot of regulars helping out. Removable ceiling tiles are often found in hospitals and other public buildings. They make marvelous canvases, because they're a manageable size and can readily be taken down, replaced, then put back up when completed. They can be mounted almost anywhere. This project also gets the hospital maintenance staff involved, because they have to help with taking them down and then replacing the tiles once they're painted. So if you're a *regular* at your hospital, or a resident at a nursing home or rehabilitation facility, and you're fit and ambulant enough, talk to the staff and your companions about starting such a project.

Jewelry and ornaments are easy to make too, using Fimo clay or Sculpey. You can attach or embed beads, colored glass pieces, lace, string, and coins to the clay to make jewels from among your collection of found art objects. Once you've softened the clay in your fingers and palms, it can be molded into any shape your heart desires. It's warm and malleable to handle, and very comforting to work with, even if you suffer from arthritis, or your hands and wrists are not as strong as they used to be. As you may know, working with these materials has long been a standby for occupational therapists in helping people with joint problems, or those who have suffered strokes, to recover their strength and flexibility.

Then there's collage-making. Collages are complex images composed of pictures usually cut out from discarded magazines and pasted on cardboard. You can use postcards, newspapers, and photographs too. They can be of any size and shape. Collages cost almost nothing, are very easy to create, supply an endless variety of visual images, and will always whet your appetite for more.

All these activities are very simple stuff, and they're great to work and play with in a support group. It just takes a little *chutzpah* to get started—that and the permission serious illness and other life-changing events give you to slow down and take a look around at the passing moment. Give yourself permission to start filling these moments with creativity and image-making.

Story: The Clinic Studio

I run a weekly outpatient clinic for my patients. They vary in age from babies to young adults, and they're almost always accompanied by a family member, most often a parent. These young people have serious life-limiting illnesses, like cancer and sickle cell disease. There's a room next to the nurses' work station where the patients can gather together, with or without their families, while they're waiting to be seen by one of the staff, or while their IVs are dripping with that day's dose of medicine or maybe a blood transfusion. There are many artists, students, and other volunteers who come to help, to learn another aspect of the healing arts, and to simply enjoy sharing time with these feisty and fun-loving young people.

This family room is now wall-to-wall and wall-to-ceiling images. They jump out at you from all directions as you enter the doorway: paintings and drawings and collages of every size and shape and color. Recently the contributors to this art gallery have had to spread themselves out into the corridor, since Lisa, the senior volunteer artist and a trained child life worker, started a new project. Her new project involves cutting out the shapes of people's bodies while they lie on a large piece of blank paper stretched on the floor. This, as you can imagine, is an uproarious process for one and all. Now there's a whole passageway lined with a fast-growing family of vividly painted, life-size paper people. They seem to be steadily streaming along the walls, hand in hand and laughing as they go. It's sort of the hospital's version of a wax museum, but all the figures are in loving connection with each other.

Exercise: Creating Collages

Let's try a collage exercise that has the added advantage of giving you something to do with your old magazines. All you'll need are four things: a pile of magazines, a pair of scissors, a glue stick for paper-pasting, and a bunch of cardboard. A highlighter can be useful too.

This is especially good fun with others. Gather around a table together, or have visitors to your hospital room bring the supplies. You'll find it's a marvelous way to doodle—to make spontaneous images, but this time using ready-made photographs. It also gets rid of that competitive edge and the feeling you might fail in full view of everyone else (or of yourself). How can you grade anyone for the pieces they chop out of a magazine and choose to put together?

Your composites can be of any size and shape you choose: there are no rules about this. And your blends of people and ads, scenery and machinery—all kinds of everyday images and situations—will add up to marvelous stories to weave back and forth with each other. Many times you'll surprise yourself with the *serendipity* of the things that suggest themselves to you; you'll end up with a nice mix-and-match of pictures culled from assorted sources. You can make up endless stories and funny anecdotes from these collages. The remarkable thing about them, though, is that the stories the collages suggest to you are rarely made up. Even without your conscious intention, you'll find within them your own story, or some piece of it, be it tragedy or comedy, thriller or high farce.

It's a good idea to spend the first ten minutes idling through your pile of magazines. The more diverse in subject they are, the better. Let the images play on your eye as you turn down the corner of a page here, highlight or ring with your pencil or highlighter a subject there. When you have about twenty subjects or pieces, go back and cut them all out. Don't worry about being too precise with the margins—let them waver and zigzag if it suits you. Now you've already got a fascinating juxtaposition of material to work with. They'll be all sizes, so pick out about half a dozen, either at random or more carefully if something suggests itself to you.

Now cut out a piece of cardboard. Again, don't worry what shape or size it is, but make it easily manageable. It should be between four inches and a foot in diameter to start with, although you can certainly take on much larger projects once you get the feel of it. Then all you're going to do is paste your magazine cutouts in any order and arrangement you choose onto your cardboard. It's best if you paste the larger pieces on first, because otherwise you might cover up the smaller bits entirely. But you don't have to worry about *partly* superimposing one on another; that's part of the design. If you're working with others, as I hope you are, I suggest you pass them around after a while, so you each get to work on several pieces. This creates a lot of fun, sort of like the mad hatter's tea party.

Now sit back and admire your handiwork. What do you see? What has appeared as you've united all these seemingly unrelated fragments? Anything—or anyone—you know? What does it trigger? Do any memories come up? Are any feelings surfacing, either happy or sad? Is there a story (or stories) here? Take a moment to reflect on how little time you spent in the last half hour or so worrying about your medical diagnosis, your life situation, what the doctor told you yesterday, or what medical tests you'll have to undergo tomorrow. You were just too busy making pictures together. Making stuff up. . . .

Story: Ellie Triages

Collage-making is an especially easy and relaxing way to make use of visual images. One of our program's professional artists-in-residence, Ellie, uses it to come down and get herself ready for sleep after she's been painting all day and half the night and is really high, or in the flow. But I guess the professional artist never really goes off duty. When this trick doesn't work and she still can't settle down, she's made a habit of taking herself off to the hospital at three or four in the morning with her easel and paints. She sets herself up in a corner of the waiting room outside the emergency room proper and starts making sketches of the people there. Some of them may have been there for hours waiting to be triaged. This is the word used in busy ERs, or at a road accident site where there's a lot of injuries, when one of the nursing or medical staff makes a quick assessment of each person to decide the priority in attending to their needs.

One night Ellie was just setting up her easel when an obviously agitated young man came in. He was pacing about the waiting room wringing his hands, wild-eyed and moaning to himself. He didn't seem to have any physical injury though, and was almost certainly suffering from what's called in medical parlance a panic attack, a state of extreme anxiety. Ellie watched him for a few minutes, then felt moved to paint his picture. After a few minutes the man became aware of her attention and seemed to quiet down a bit. Before much longer, he moved over to take a look at what she was up to. As he did so, and she continued to depict him on her canvas, he became more and more absorbed in what she was producing—the image of himself. With his absorption he grew calmer and calmer. When she was done, she tore off the picture and handed it to him. He promptly announced that he was feeling fine now, and left the premises without even registering his name with the clerk!

I think it was the concentrated attention that Ellie showed to him as a fellow human being that must have done the trick. Perhaps he saw in the picture something in which he could take pride, and this brought him back to the reality of his situation: that he was really okay, and didn't need any medical intervention. Such is the power of art and artists.

Your Personal Mandala

Ellie has a particularly fun way of making collages. She finds combinations of images—maybe only two cutouts—for a collage that tells a definite story. Or else she juxtaposes two images on a postcard that together create a hilarious situation; it's visual joke-telling. Collage-making can be used more seriously too. Mary Lisa, the artist coordinator at Shands Hospital in Gainesville, Florida since 1993, works with groups of patients, medical students, and staff making *mandala collages*.

The word *mandala* is Sanskrit for "wheel." It is a mostly circular image with a central focal point. It's derived from Indian and Tibetan religious tradition, and is often used as a centering symbol for prayer. These sacred circles of art-making have become a cornerstone of the modern discipline of art therapy. Jung found them a valuable aid in his psychotherapy and creative healing practice. Mary Lisa uses them more freely than in this somewhat ritualistic format, but still with a serious purpose: that of taking a look at yourself, and telling yourself and your companions your story. You can even use mandala-making for *seeing* or planning your future.

Collage-making lends itself well to the creation of mandalas. Try going through your magazine collection again, but this time with a particular theme in mind. It may be your illness, your life situation, your family, or perhaps the year ahead. Try choosing just those images that *feel* as if they have a particular significance to your theme. If you pay good attention and look and listen well, certain images that you come across may even seem to be calling to you to be chosen: "Come on, pick me, pick me."

This is your intuition at play, the heart and soul of giving your imagination and creativity free reign in your art-making. This is how you and I and all of us can happen upon *the truth of the imagination*. This isn't just John Keats' but every artist's version of the truth: It's no less true for not having a rational basis or explanation. I remember an artist's response to someone who asked her rather skeptically what evidence she had that art healed anything or anyone: "I have the evidence of my instincts and my intuition, backed up by twenty years of observing with an artist's eye. That's the evidence I have." As if to say, Hey mister, d'you have any problem with that? Such evidence is in its authentic way as good as any scientific proof.

Exercise: Making Your Personal Mandala

Use another big blank sheet of paper for this. (You can use cardboard instead if you want to make it sturdier for display, or mount your paper version after it's completed.) You'll need your box of wax crayons or chalk pastels, whichever you've found works best for you. That's it. That's all you'll need. Spread yourself and your art supplies out on your table, floor, bed.

Once more, take a little time to let go of any feelings you may have about "not being an artist." We all have to perform that little ritual repeatedly, so you're in good company. None of these exercises ever has anything to do with how *good* a picture you can create. It may help you to think of the word "good" in one of its other meanings, two of which are "virtuous" and "loving." That's not a lot to ask of all these new friends you've created—that they help you appreciate how full of goodness and loving virtue you are.

Okay, shake out all your crayons or chalks from the box. Does this remind you of anything? Do you remember the last time you did this? Played with chalks or crayons in such an assortment of colors? It may well have been a few years. Just take a look at them all, and see their marvelous variety. Last time I limited you to using just one or two colors that seemed to choose you. This time I give you permission to use every one of your forty-eight Crayolas if you want to!

Now all you have to do is draw one large circle on your blank surface. Be sure to make it a good size, because within this space you've created you're going to put *yourself*. More exactly, you're going to fill this space with several aspects of yourself as you see them. Your physical self, your mental self, and your emotional self, your spiritual self, and yourself in relation to others and to your environment. These are the six dimensions of yourself that have to do with health. They're all linked within you, and they're all equally important, not any one more so than any other.

Now you can use any of these colors that catch your fancy. You don't need to obey the rules, because there are no rules here. The point is not to create literal and precise representations, but rather to capture images of how you see these different bits of you. In other words, how do you *imagine* the state of health of your body-mind-spirit at the moment? How healthy are your relationships to other people, and to this beloved planet we all inhabit together?

Please notice, if you haven't already, that with mandalas there is no *right* place on the paper to start, no top left-hand corner. Just jump in wherever you want to—and with whatever comes to you first. In fact, it's important not to think ahead too much. Try to keep this as easy and spontaneous as you can. This is *not* an exercise for your logical left brain, but for your inventive right brain. You may just want to play with shades of light and dark, rather than with any recognizable objects to represent you. But by all means draw yourself as a stick figure or a balloon body, then add the bits of yourself you want in there. Even dare to throw in a few bits that you don't like too much, or that you don't really want cluttering things up. They're significant too, perhaps especially so.

You don't have to fill every nook and cranny of your sacred circle. Nor do you actually have to stay strictly within it. Venturing over the lines—a little irreverently—may suit your style or mood. So use the colors to express your personality, and to speak to the state of health of each part of yourself. If you find your circle isn't big enough just start another one on a new sheet: "You—Part 2," you might call it. You can of course devote a mandala to each dimension of yourself. A whole sketchbook full of different parts of you is not a bad notion at all.

Your Intuitive Intelligence at Work

Now you've had a chance to make your own mandala. This is one way art can help you tell your story and so get a greater understanding of yourself, and it's another project you can put down and pick up again as often as you like, just as the spirit moves you. It's good to put your self-mandala away and come back to it after a rest. Return to it in new versions as you become aware of aspects of your health that you haven't paid too much attention to. Take a look-see.

What have you said about yourself? What part of your intuitive intelligence was at work when you weren't watching?

That's the way it works with art, and even with science too. Albert Einstein, the greatest scientific genius of the twentieth century, used to wonder why he got all his best ideas while he was shaving in the morning after a twelve-hour sleep. But he also acknowledged that this was why he slept so much—because it was during sleep that he got the *real* work done, when his imagination was going full tilt in his dreams. Imagination, he said, was more important than knowledge.

Dreams and Art-Making

Which brings us to dream-making. Dreams are at the very heart of your imaginative genius. Some people say they never dream, but the scientific evidence suggests that every human being dreams deeply and widely whenever they sleep. It's just that many remember only disjointed fragments or nothing at all. Carl Jung saw human beings as undergoing dreams—as being their recipients or objects—just as if dreams visited us from unknown, or barely acknowledged, spiritual realms. Christina Baldwin puts it in her book *Life's Companion: Journal Writing as a Spiritual Quest* (1991 p. 137) like this: "We are both the dreamer and the dreamed."

Your dreams are pure symbol and metaphor: a continuous work of art. You can call them inner movies if you like. They also represent the most pressing of your life's problems and puzzles that you need to resolve, because you're constantly in your waking life assigning yourself such homework, to take out and study once you're in bed asleep. Dreams contain within them many possible answers to your questions and quests: They can be your guide and counselor. As I said earlier, dreams were a central part of the healing ceremonies of the priests and priestesses of the temples of Delphi and Epidarus in ancient Greece.

Exercise: Re-creating Your Dreams

This exercise needs to be done upon waking from sleep. I've adapted it from several used in Christina Baldwin's book. You'll need your pen or your colored pencils, together with your workbook or journal (although people who record their dreams regularly keep a special dream journal). It's important to keep your journal and at least a pen or pencil by your bedside. Everyone has had the experience of waking from a rich dream, only to have it already escape into the stratosphere by the time you've completed a couple of bathroom activities. So try to get into the habit of writing descriptions of your dreams as soon as you wake, even when you wake up during the night.

As you come out of sleep, bring your mind to immediate present consciousness by staying still and breathing quietly and deeply. Pick up your pen and workbook. At once begin to write down the images or story that you can capture from whatever was going on in your dream the moment before waking. This often takes some practice, especially if you are one of those who thinks they never dream, or never remember their dreams. Persevere for several days; it will be worth it. If you're in the habit of taking daytime naps—and everyone should—you can use these as more occasions for dream-recording.

Use phrases or even single words and simple drawings to depict what you've just experienced or imagined in your dream. Record everything in the *present tense*, as though you're redreaming it. This will help you reenter and relive your dream. You don't need grammatically correct sentences. Move quickly, jotting down a few words and images to capture the essence. Try to catch what seem to be the most significant or recurring objects or symbols. Your dream may be joyful and comforting, or stressful and even terrifying. But try not to duck anything or leave anything out. Once you've gotten going, try using your colored pencils or crayons for writing words or drawing pictures to represent the dream's content. You'll find it quite easy to choose the *right* colors for different symbolic objects, people, or activities in your dream.

Now take another page and see if you can compose all you've recorded in words and pictures into a story line. Talk to your dream's characters; ask them who they are and what they want of you. Go on drawing and writing as the answers come to you. Always remember that nothing has to make rational sense at first, but accept that everything is important. Some clear guidance and answers are likely to come if you persist with this habit.

Come back to this dream exercise often, even daily, as a way to deepen and enrich your art-making. Your dreams are also your friends, even when they give you symbolic messages that frighten you or that you don't want to hear.

Process and Product

I hope you've already had the idea of decorating your room, or the space you've set aside for your artistic activities, with some of your "finished products" of visual art. I put this phrase in quotes because actually no work of art that you create need ever be finished. It's all process.

If you do use your work for decoration, you'll quickly see how putting a bunch of bits and pieces on a wall, or stringing them up across the room with paste, or with needle and thread on a string like holiday cards, transforms the space. Even if each fragment of work has little intrinsic merit to your judgmental eye, look at what a work of art you can create by pulling several of these fragments into a group or collage to create a *whole piece*. If you're in a hospital room or a nursing home, imagine how much more interesting your space is going to be to staff and visitors. You'll probably get a lot more—and more enjoyable—visits.

Displaying Your Work

It's well worth being thoughtful about what you place where. As I've told you, the Chinese astrological art of feng shui has been used for millennia as a guide to how to arrange the immediate environment step by step for optimal balance and harmony, or the flow of chi. You can do this too: You don't have to hail from ancient China. There are several excellent books written for Western lay people on this subject, for example those by T. Raphael Simons (1996) and William Spear (1995), that will tell you a great deal about feng shui and your health. As Simons points out, your state of mind and energy affect your environment for good or bad, while the condition of your environment in turn influences your internal state of mind and spirit. All you need do is use your attention, your intuition, and a little knowledge, to accommodate every aspect of your life in a single space. It's easy to get a small space cluttered, overfurnished, and overdecorated.

As these images you're creating grow and spread, they will feed off each other. If you give yourself the permission, you'll find yourself coming up with more and more ideas, diversion, inspiration, and comfort. In our hospital's atrium stands what is called the Healing Wall. It consists of about 1200 six-inch-by-six-inch ceramic tiles. Each one was painted by a patient or family member, a staff member or student. No one of them has enormous artistic merit, although many have great significance in their content and symbolism. But when Leanne, the artist who conceptualized this work, put them all together, it was as though suddenly there appeared a transcendent work of art. The collected images of so many people, drawn together by the challenge, the tragedy, and even the rewards of illness, beckon you timelessly to draw near, in homage, love, admiration, and worship.

Our Healing Wall is very reminiscent of the AIDS quilt, which was first displayed in Washington, D.C. in 1987. This quilt contains twenty-thousand panels, each with a name and tribute to someone who has died of AIDS. It has become a vital artistic and spiritual symbol of universal love and support, facilitating both mourning and healing for a whole community, that of gay men, who at that time had been shunned by the rest of society when the disease started to spread among them.

Art-Making as Friend and Ally

So ... how are you doing? Still daunted by the very idea of painting? Still shy about displaying your creations for all to see? Or are you finding yourself taken up with this process, with this ritual of lifting paints or crayons or chalks or modeling clay from the box, starting a new piece on a new sheet or canvas, or coming back to the one you put aside last night? Are you feeling just a little pride and satisfaction at giving your art-making instinct full rein? Are you perhaps getting a bit excited at the thought of working some more on your new project, getting reacquainted with your *new friend*?

Are you even noticing yourself more in charge of your surroundings, of your situation? Are you feeling more supported, less intimidated and overwhelmed, less out of control and helpless? Because as you call upon your new skills as friends and supporters to cheer you up and cheer you on, you might very well find yourself *thinking* more clearly as well as *feeling* more healthy. You may find yourself able to frame your thoughts more succinctly, and knowing immediately what questions you want to ask of your doctor, what your priorities are, and what decisions you have to make. And you may find yourself more committed to making them.

Art-making does this for you. This is its power. It's the work of the right brain in service to the left. Art is never idle. While you sleep, and the images scamper and scuttle about in your subconscious— playing with your unprotesting mind, forming new images and symbols—they will suggest a thousand new ways to look at your situation. Art will guide you in which direction you should turn to achieve your greatest health and your truest destiny. A higher awareness will have begun to arouse from its long slumber within you, albeit still unconscious to your waking self.

It will if you let it start to take charge of your present and future fortune once more, in the straightforward, unerringly accurate way of the very young. You just may be catching some sure-footed glimpses of your authentic self. You may be becoming once more the child who still remembers heaven.

But you have to listen. And watch—with your inner ear and eye.

5

Words Read,
Words Said

Inside every patient there's a poet trying to get out.

—Anatole Broyard

Stories of Home: Narrative Psychology

Remember how in the opening chapter Don the pastor used story-telling as a way to draw people together? The patients were spending Thanksgiving in the hospital, many of them far from home, at the very time of year in our country when home is what people yearn for most, symbolically and literally. But the next best thing is to revisit your home in memory and in story, to use your imagination to recapture sights and sounds and smells and feels. After all, there's no place like it, as Dorothy in *The Wizard of Oz* reminded us.

Home may have some unhappy associations for you too, from which you longed to escape. But for all of us it represents something closest to our authentic selves, nearest to where we *belong*. Accepting its constraints and conflicts, as well as celebrating the nurturance and security it gives us, are mental activities common to everyone. Who hasn't had dreams of one or more of the homes they've lived in? My friend and colleague Gail Ellison wrote a whole Ph.D. dissertation (1996) on house dreams as symbols of illness and recovery. She explored the many ways in which people *use* such dreams of houses they've lived in as a way of wrestling with issues both of getting ill and of coming to full health once more.

Gail's work falls into the category of narrative psychology, because it explores how human beings use words continuously to tell stories as a means to better emotional health—through conversations and letters, journal writing and poetry, on up to novels, memoirs, and autobiographies. In this chapter I'll offer you some ways you can polish up the fine art of words. I hope you'll come to not only enjoy their more creative use, but through this particular form of art-making come to feel both more generally healthy and also able to think more clearly about your life situation and what you need to do next.

Exercise: "Scoffs and Scorns and Contumelious Taunts"

The title of this exercise is a Shakespearean quote that translates into modern parlance as "put-downs." Because many of us have a lifetime of discouragement behind us when we set out to be creative and do things differently from the norm, I'll continue to urge you to act the rebel and free yourself from such negativity. I've adapted this exercise from one in *A Creative Companion* (1991) by SARK. It's wonderful for releasing tension, dismissing doubts, and promoting creativity. All you'll need is your workbook and a pen or pencil, a paper or plastic bag, and a rubber band or piece of string.

Take a fresh page of your workbook and give yourself five minutes of writing time. You're going to write down every single word you can think of—every one you've *ever* heard—that has any put-down connotation. I'll start you off with a few you can copy down: hopeless, cynical, daunting, silly, mocking, sarcastic, derisive, sneering, stupid, smart-alecky, caustic . . . and so on. Let your mind run on from there.

Keep going for five minutes. Fill as much of one sheet as you can with all these discouraging words. When your time's up, tear out the page from your workbook and rip it up into as many shreds as you can. Really get into this part with vigor; you should be quite breathless at the end of it. Then you're going to stuff all these shreds of put-down words into your paper or plastic bag and seal it at the top with a rubber band or tie it with a piece of string. Make it so you can shape the bag into the rough shape of a soccer ball, because here comes another fun part: You get to kick this ball of *dirty words* around the floor for as long as you have the energy to do so. You can even accompany your kicks with a few yells of rejoicing. Try shouting out some self-affirming phrases like "I'm done with you!", "Ah, free at last!", "The real me!", and so on. Once you're done with kicking and screaming (or instead, if this is a bit too energetic for you, simply drumming your fists up and down on it), make a ceremony out of tossing your bag of put-downs into the garbage can. There—it's history.

Story: Sarah the Ward Clerk

We had a clerk on one of our hospital's inpatient units, whom I'll call Sarah. Clerks are responsible for a vast variety of duties and activities: answering every telephone call, keeping the patient census current and correct, filing all that paperwork in the charts, ordering up every kind of supply, dispatching patient orders to Pharmacy and the patients themselves to X-ray or the OR, and so on and on. No modern hospital unit could function without these enormously efficient and often underappreciated beings. They have no direct patient care responsibilities but many ward clerks somehow find time to get to know the longer-stay patients, offering a listening ear in times of trouble. Right in the center of the ward's comings and goings, not much escapes them. Sarah was one of those who went above and beyond.

She was always a spiritual woman, something of a lay preacher. On the unit where she worked there were many ill patients, and not a few deaths. In the nature of things, word would quickly get around that there'd been a death during the night. Morale would sometimes be low, not only among the patients and families but also their caregivers. I made a habit of checking in with Sarah each morning before my rounds, to take the temperature of the day—how things were not only with her, but with everyone else I'd be encountering. She could always give me an accurate read on the mood of things.

Sometimes we had time to talk a little more together; on those occasions she'd recount a story of a patient from some time back whom I'd forgotten about. I realized she knew more about some of my patients than I did, especially about their family lives. These were the little stories she'd hear as they paused at her desk, or as she was delivering supplies to their room. She never told me anything clearly confidential between them and herself, although she would share stories with me of patients who had passed on—tales I would otherwise never have heard. I came to the realization that it wasn't just her accessibility that made her the confidante for so many over such a long period. Her brief anecdotes were always full of tenderness, praise, compassion, and love for all those less fortunate.

I took to listening in on some of the more unguarded exchanges at the nurses' station where Sarah held sway. What came through clearly was her unconscious and quite untrained skill with words. She had ways of appreciating and acknowledging everyone, instantly seeing another's situation and viewpoint—skills of which any professional counselor would be justly proud. Sarah was a natural artist in *healing with words.*

Exercise: Splitting Story-Time

This is an exercise for sharing with one other person. You're going to trade stories of home, past and present, just as did those patients on the cancer ward. It doesn't matter whom you choose, as long as it's someone you like to spend time with. A spouse or close friend, a fellow patient or staff member if you're in the hospital: any one of these is perfect.

You won't need tools or equipment, only a little quiet, undisturbed time together. Twenty minutes will be fine, but the longer the better. Get yourselves settled, as close together as is comfy. You're going to split whatever time you've assigned to this exercise evenly in two, so decide who will tell his story first. The essential thing to realize is that this isn't simply back-and-forth conversation. Like the check-in ritual you did earlier, it's about really listening to each other deeply, quietly, and uninterruptedly. Which means no "Oh yes, that reminds me of . . . ," nor even allowing your own thoughts to stray from the other person's story, if he brings up something that triggers a memory in you. This is *his* time, and then it'll be *your* time. So note the time right now and begin.

It makes sense to start with your current home, painting a word-picture of its size and appearance, what you like most about it, and where you like to spend your leisure hours. Also say something about who shares your home with you: partner, children, pets, plants. How long have you lived there? How did you find it, and what was it about it that first attracted you? Was it love at first sight, or were there some real compromises with your heart's desire? Do you know anything about the people who lived there before you?

Conjure up some of your favorite memories of life there. Let this lead on to other memories of other homes. Recapture the sights and sounds, and especially the smells and feels, as best you can. Smells are particularly evocative of early times. They will often take you back to your first beginnings in life if you let them. What are some of the colors you've always used to decorate your home? Are there pieces of furniture you've carried from place to place? What does thinking about that old couch or kitchen table bring up for you? Don't be afraid to let some of the sad memories surface. Art, like life, is not all a bed of roses, but this is a perfect chance to share some of those tough times of being brought up, or bringing up your own children. This is a perfect place to share some of the losses every home is witness to, whether through death or school graduations that lead inexorably to empty nests. Expressing—which means literally *pushing out*—grief is a natural human behavior that we too often feel the need to repress, like many of our emotions.

Soon enough it will be time to trade places. When you're listening to the other person's story, just drop quietly into it with all your antennae out. Listen deeply and see in your mind's eye the pictures that her words offer you. Because in the time together that this exercise affords you, you have the equal joy of making your own trips down memory lane, and *also* having a story—or a dream, or a vision—of someone else's home to sink into.

Once both your times are up, pause for a moment and linger silently and companionably over these stories you've re-created together. Breathe in the memories once more. You'll probably have jarred loose all kinds of other ones that you didn't have time to share. But like all the exercises in this book, you can revisit it as often as you like. If you want to and have the time, just recheck your watch and start over right now. But remember an essential final rule: You should treat anything that your partner has shared with you as confidential, just as you can expect your partner to treat your story in the same way. This an essential rule for any ritual exchange of this kind. It creates the necessary safety that makes this a truly heartfelt sharing.

Journaling for Health

This doesn't of course stop you from writing notes in your workbook, or your journal, of all your own memories, thoughts, and feelings that may have come up during this time together. Like all the healing arts, the art of journal writing has taken an upturn in popularity recently. Not only are more and more people turning to journaling, it has also been the subject of many medical and psychological studies, as I'll go into a bit later. Not only are people turning to it individually, but writing groups are also springing up in every community, often more with the goal of mutual support than in order to get one's writing published.

Two of my favorite books about such personal writing are Christina Baldwin's *Life's Companion: Journal Writing as a Spiritual Quest* (1991) and Julia Cameron's *The Artist's Way* (1992). As its name implies, Christina Baldwin's book is concerned with making a spiritual journey, which she sees as one we're all on together, whether with awareness or, more often, without it. It could be a valuable resource if you or a loved one are dealing with serious illness. As she points out, everyone needs a map for making a journey, and writing your journal can help you make a map of your life: past, present, and future. Her book is a delight to read; it's full of easy exercises, meditations, and quotations.

Julia Cameron's book is much broader in scope, but also concerned with a spiritual path to recovering your creative self. One of her basic tools for this purpose is what she calls *the morning pages*. These are simply three pages of longhand writing that she instructs you to complete every day—strictly *stream of consciousness*. This means absolutely no preparing, no thinking about what you're writing, and most of all no censoring any thought or word. This exercise consists of just moving your pen automatically across the page. She credits this simple—she even calls it meaningless—exercise with helping many people recover their artistic selves from wherever they'd last seen them, perhaps way back in their childhoods. In trying this you may well find, just as she tells you to expect, that the first couple of pages are pretty dull. But by page three you'll start to uncover something meatier about your current situation.

Exercise: *Writing the Wrongs*

You just did an exercise in which you split time with a friend or family member, telling something of your early or recent memories of how home has been and what it has meant to you. So you're well warmed up for this next one. You're going to write a brief but fairly comprehensive story of your life.

Storytelling is as old as human speech. In ancient times, it took place wherever people came together: at the well to gather water or the riverside to wash clothes, around the campfire after a hunt or battle. Today storytelling seems to be more confined to the priest's confessional or psychologist's couch. But the deliberate telling of your tale is a good way to reflect on and make sense of things past, to restore through restorying yourself. It can help you uncover and face difficult truths, see things in new ways, gain perspective, and come to acceptance of your situation.

You need only your workbook or possibly a separate book you set aside as your journal, plus your favorite pen or pencil. It can be helpful (and fun too) to have a look around for any old photos you may have at home to jog your memories. Taking a fresh page, write the numbers 1 to 10 down the left-hand side, one per line. Then continue on down each line with every other number: 12, 14, 16, 18, 20. Then continue to the bottom and over to the next page if need be with every fifth number: 25, 30, 35, 40, and so on. Continue in this sequence until you reach your current age.

You're going to write a short sentence—a few words will do— on each line, to describe something about each of these years of your life. You'll end up with something about each year of the first ten, stretching it to two-year spells as a teenager, and to five-year periods during your adult years. Don't think too hard though, and if you really can't recall anything from your earliest years, make something up that you think may well have happened.

This may take you twenty minutes, but don't take longer than that. You can come back to it to fill in the blanks. You'll be amazed how you'll jog free some memories that you thought were long since buried. Once you've got your list of lines, go over them to see how many have a positive and how many a negative slant. Because this is called "Writing the Wrongs," I want you to choose one line that has a bad memory for you, or at least not a happy one. You're going to expand on the few words you wrote.

Thinking of those words, start to *free-write*, without pause for thought, whatever comes into your mind. Who was in your life at that time? What were your circumstances? Where were you living? What about it is hard or painful to remember? As your hand moves across the page, let yourself be aware of it, and of the flow of ink from your pen, as a way of keeping yourself in touch with the reality of your presence here today. Just because you're revisiting a sad or painful memory doesn't mean you're literally going back there. Keeping half an eye—and part of your mind—on the safe and sound present moment serves as a constant reminder of this. Remember too that no one else need ever read what you're writing, unless you choose. You can say anything you like: Put it out there, and if it's a hurtful memory, remind yourself as often as you need to that it's all past history, which has no power over you anymore.

Story: Curt's Family Diary

Curt's a nurse I've known for ten years. He's about my age, and although we don't work on the same hospital unit, we often bump into each other. I found out he had an interest in art too, and he got interested in our Arts in Medicine program in the hospital. A skilled amateur photographer, he would come and take pictures when we put on workshops or brought in performing artists for special occasions.

One day he told me he'd started keeping a journal. This was something he'd done occasionally as a young man, but he'd put it aside for many years. What precipitated his taking it up again was his mother's illness. He'd moved his seventy-six-year-old mom up from south Florida so he could look after her after his father died. He was worried she couldn't fend well for herself—a fear that proved only too well founded. A month after she'd moved in she started having memory lapses and episodes of confusion, particularly at night. Once he found her wandering down the middle of the street in her nightie. The neurologist confirmed the diagnosis: Alzheimer's disease, with a rather rapid and unrelenting course.

Curt is a single parent whose seventeen-year-old son and thirteen-year-old daughter live with him. He has a steady job as a nurse that pays quite well, but he knew he needed help, which he'd have to pay for, in order to keep his mother out of a nursing home. He very much wanted to put this off, and if possible avoid it for good. "Things got pretty wild for a while. Myself and two other generations living in a small three-bedroom house, all more or less dependent on me for livelihood and attention. My children are great kids and help a lot, but I can't turn them into long-term babysitters to their grandma."

Curt couldn't afford a full-time live-in nurse, and he even contemplated going half-time at work so he could spend more time with his mother. Although he had a lot of friends, he was reluctant to call on them, perhaps out of pride and a reluctance to feel obligated. His journal became his live-in friend, his ally.

"As my mom got progressively more unpredictable in her behavior, especially in her sleeping patterns, I took to sitting up with my journal after she and the kids were bedded down, sometimes into the small hours. I soon found myself kind of 'chatting' with my journal, like it was an old army buddy. It was really comforting. I'd been dating occasionally up till then, but I didn't feel safe about leaving mom alone, and I didn't feel like bringing dates home. Things were crowded enough already. And I guess I was embarrassed about her. She'd have bouts of swearing like a trooper, and sometimes she'd start taking her clothes off in the kitchen and so on.

"So I'd simply write. And write some more. Mostly without thinking much about the words I was putting down on the page. It was quite a scrawl—I certainly didn't have to worry about anyone else reading it! Then I realized what my mind—my instincts—were up to: I, or they, were just wanting to get some perspective on things, and this seemed to be the best way to do it. To take stock of everything, and make plans on paper. Then more and more I found myself fishing up old memories of home, times with Mom and Dad and my younger brother. I'd gotten pretty lonely, and I'd often cry for a while over 'the good old days.' I'm still pissed at my ex too, and I was having a bunch of trouble with her about how I was handling Matt." (Matt was the seventeen-year-old who'd moved from his mom's house the year before after a series of school truancy and other problems.) "So my buddy, as I came to call 'him,' was party to a lot of bitching about the whole set-up. I'd always been a pretty easygoing sort, so I was amazed at all the rage and colorful language that was coming up. It felt pretty good actually.

"So I wrote a lot. I filled a couple of looseleaf notebooks in the first month or so after Mom moved in. Well, the thing I noticed after a few weeks was that I'd started to feel a lot better. A whole lot calmer. I really looked forward to 'seeing' my buddy each night. Almost like a date! I suppose a journal is a kind of love affair. All those confidences, sharing myself in a way I'd never done with anyone in fifty-odd years. I used to be able to talk to Mom when I was a little kid, and even after I got to college—probably more than most sons and moms. So it was really sad that I couldn't get through to her any more about my stuff.

"Actually that's not fair. She used to have pretty good days—not nowadays much at all, but for the first year maybe. Then we'd have real fun. Would you believe she liked to play table tennis when she was in high school—I never knew. I don't know where she got the notion—maybe from the TV, but she told me one day she wanted to play. Just like that. So I got a table top that fits on the dining room table and all the equipment. She remembered it immediately, after sixty years or so. Amazing. Uncanny really, when already most days she didn't know where she was. She doesn't want to do it much anymore—she's too far gone—but she and my daughter and I play some nights and weekends. Just great. We're getting pretty good!

"The thing about this whole journal thing is that I noticed after a bit that I was able to settle down and get to sleep soundly afterwards, and I'd wake up feeling better, really relaxed. I was able to think much more clearly about things too, in a more problem-solving way. They say a good cry or a good tantrum clears your head. Well, this way of expressing myself certainly worked for me. In some ways I've been happier this past year than for a long time. I've got a lot of purpose to my life, I'm staying out of the bars, and I'm getting pretty close to the kids. I've managed to keep Mom at home, even though I know most folks—men anyway—would have given up and packed her off to some kind of facility a while back. I don't know how it's going to end up, but I think I've done pretty damn well so far. And I really think my journal-buddy can take a lot of credit."

A New Social Service

When people get sick, their family members often have a harder time than the sick person. This has never been more true than in the case of Alzheimer's disease, where a loved one's mind is failing progressively before your eyes. This is not to suggest that the affected person doesn't suffer—especially in the early days when they still have insight into the problem, and are aware of themselves gradually losing their grip on things. But looking on in helpless witness of such deterioration, whether it be physical or mental, carries its own particularly painful burden of suffering. This is the legacy, for both the affected one and those near and dear, of chronic illness that progresses without relief.

Many illnesses and disabilities, like diabetes or a stroke, are chronic but stay fairly stable for years. However, there are some, particularly neurological or blood problems, that follow this inexorable course, and all the nearest and dearest can do is watch powerlessly. The medical profession, not having much to offer, doesn't feel it can fill its offices and hospital clinics with these folks, when doctors have little or nothing to treat them with. Managed care companies place strict limits on reimbursement as well. So these patients and their families can feel more or less on their own, apart from the aid of some social services. And these services are pretty spotty in many places, especially in the face of recent widespread cutbacks.

Curt chanced on a *social service* that no one could ever cut back on—except himself, if he ever chose to. It would always be there for him, more faithful than a hound dog to its master. And indeed he is its master, as we are of anything we create entirely ourselves. But such a creation, or work of art, seems to take on its own personality and spirit, as you'll quickly discover when you try it for yourself. Because make no mistake about it, a journal is a work of art, of inspired creation. And your journal is always there for you: to be of service to you at all times, like all the best servants. It will always offer you an intently listening ear, and be brimming with friendly counsel. It will always be watching out for your best interests, if you listen well enough to what it's saying to you.

Journals: The Research

So here's yet another area in which you have complete mastery. Journaling, or spontaneous personal writing, means just about anything that isn't technical or scientific (or a shopping list). It is writing that comes out of your own memories and stories, perhaps enhanced by your dreams, wishes, and imagination. It's especially comforting at times when everything seems to be going to hell in a handcart, and you have no apparent control over anything. Countless people have tried putting pen or pencil to their journal books—or to the backs of envelopes or other scraps—and found for themselves the value of talking on paper. If you thought that people who talked to themselves were crazy, let me reassure you it's not so: They may be among the sanest.

The evidence from scientific studies on the health-promoting effects of keeping a regular diary is compelling. The best-known researcher in this field of creative writing is Dr. James Pennebaker, a psychologist at Southern Methodist University. He has distilled much of his work into a book for lay people called *Opening Up: The Healing Power of Confiding in Others* (1997). The title is misleading. Although as a psychologist he has used the time-honored methods of client/ therapist dialogue both clinically and in his research on confession, or opening up, his unique contribution is to put journal writing on the map scientifically. He has used carefully designed methods for studying this art, and has shown that telling your story on paper has a powerfully beneficial effect on your health. And it isn't just on your emotional and mental health, but on your physical and social health too.

Dr. Pennebaker, along with others, has concentrated particularly on the process of writing about traumatic events that may still haunt you from your past. The benefit seems to come from the potent links between your central nervous system and immune system. It's in line with Dr. Ader's theories of psychoneuroimmunology that I told you about earlier. The health benefits don't seem to be limited to any particular medical disorder either, and work as well with "healthy" as with "ill" people. The general observation everyone agrees with is that holding back or repressing your thoughts and feelings is hard and harmful emotional work. It eventually translates into deterioration in many aspects of your health. We all need to express, or push out into the world outside, our emotions—anger and grief, envy and fear, as well as of course joy and love. Personal writing is a simple supplement to the use of friends or therapists for fully expressing yourself. The best news of all is that it's always there and accessible. You don't have to make a date or an appointment. Many prisoners of war and those in our overcrowded jails will attest to its life-saving benefits, even if they've had to resort to scratching with their nails on their cell walls for lack of paper and pencil.

The other beautiful aspect of putting your stories on paper is that you don't have to share them with anyone else. Your *confession* can be to yourself alone. It's very hard sometimes to admit some of your thoughts and feelings even to yourself. But how much easier this is than doing so to another, even someone you trust or who is close to you. And if you don't want to even look at some of the horrid things you've written down, you can always use invisible ink. It works just as well.

Exercise: The Lost Art of Letter Writing

Journaling isn't the only type of writing that can improve your well-being. Think about this: How often do you write letters? If you're like most people, it's limited to postcards from vacation spots and notes stuck in the annual round of holiday cards to family and old friends far away. My mailbox is always full, but it contains ten items of junk mail to every handwritten letter. A hundred years ago, letter writing was a widely favored and elegant way of communicating, but in this computer age it's even earned the derisory term *snail mail*. One of the few people I know who's an avid letter writer is my friend and teacher Patch Adams. He pens hundreds every month—all longhand—to friends new and old all over the world. I don't think he's ever used a computer or word-processor, so technology glitches and computer viruses don't slow him down any.

If you have some time on your hands, how better to spend it than composing longhand letters to all those people you haven't connected with for much too long? I'm going to offer you several variations on the normal letter-writing format. You don't need to use anything other than your workbook, but if you prefer not to tear pages out of it, get yourself some standard letter-writing materials, or have someone else do so if you can't manage it yourself. There are lots of pretty letter cards and interesting postcards available that lend themselves to quite short letters. You'll need envelopes as well, and of course you'll have to make a trip to the post office for stamps.

Start by making a list of all the people you'd like to have contact with. You'll soon realize what fun this is when you come up with all the names, and start thinking of all the news you have to catch them up on. Letter writing is like journaling, in that it gives you a lot of solace and satisfaction to talk about yourself and your life on paper. But unlike journaling, you get to send letters, and with any luck receive a reply in a few days or a week or two. It's a two-way thing, like conversation. Nowadays you can trace people whose addresses you've lost through the Internet, but as you make your list, perhaps you'd like to limit your list to names in your address book. Apart from old friends and family, there may be people of recent acquaintance you'd like to write to. If you're in a hospital, why not find out from a nurse which patient has been there the longest, or gets the fewest visitors? This would be an excellent person to write to, rather like becoming a pen pal with someone who could certainly use the friendly contact.

You don't have to be far away to receive a letter; you can even be in the same room.

I suggest you write one or two a day until you've exhausted your list. By that time you should be getting replies. So that it isn't too daunting a task, keep your letters short—maybe two pages maximum—although of course you may find yourself getting really carried away with all you have to say, in which case by all means keep going. A variation on the standard letter-writing format is to write with your nondominant hand. You'll be amazed how this frees up your imagination and sense of humor. It's especially good with old friends who've known you since childhood. The same goes for your mom or dad, brothers or sisters. If they query why on earth you're doing this, tell them I told you to, and why don't they try it too? You can choose your favorite colored pen or pencil to write with, or, even better, use several colors for different sections. Illustrate it lavishly with little drawings of faces, your animals or plants or whatever takes your fancy, keeping it all easy and fun. I dare you to say you don't feel uplifted after such an exercise.

Not every letter has to be mailed. Ever heard of writing to someone you're mad at right after a fight with them, then instead of mailing it, stuffing it in a drawer for a few days or perhaps indefinitely? So you may have such a letter you want to write, especially if life has been treating you badly, and you've had a hard time getting along with a few folks. How about writing such a *no-holds-barred* letter right now?

My favorite variation on this letter-writing theme is to write a love letter—to yourself. Remember those love letters you used to write when you were a teenager. You may well have a stack of them stored in some secret place. Now I want you to compose a really gushy love letter to yourself. Once again, use your favorite pen or colored pencil, and make sure you include a lot of those favorite words of endearment. By the time you're finished, you should have at least one of each of the following: angel, love, fascinating, beauty, ecstasy, courageous, handsome, wild, funny, charm, energy, sensitive, caring, and so on. Then sprinkle it with kisses and seal it with a set of lovey-dovey initials like S.W.A.K.

The Art of Problem Solving on Paper

You should have quite a pile of letter-writing assignments by now. Most of these you'll send, and hopefully receive answers to, but some may be for you to keep in your workbook. It's the process, just as with journaling, that's the crucial thing. Letter writing—particularly to someone you care about and trust—is a lovely way to help sort out your ideas, get perspective on things, make decisions, and feel generally better about yourself.

When Dr. Pennebaker was first doing his research on therapeutic writing with his volunteer subjects, he had them write for short spells about everything from unimportant events and activities to the most heavily traumatic things in their lives to date. The significant thing he found was that it works best to put your deepest thoughts and feelings on paper, not just the facts themselves. Once you've done that, it turns out to be even more beneficial to deliberately add a problem-solving dimension. Just like any good psychotherapy session, it's most helpful if you first get things off your chest; then, when you're feeling a bit better and clearer, start thinking things through, sorting out options and making decisions, giving yourself pats on the back and other present-moment encouragement—all on paper.

This is what turns out to be the key factor in the art of writing for healing. You can have too much of a good thing. Immersing yourself in writing about yucky stuff can become as self-feeding and gratuitous as can constant complaining. The often-used phrase for this habit, which can become an addiction for some, is *awfulizing and catastrophizing.* "Ain't it awful" can certainly become a substitute for "I can do it!"—in the mind as well as the body. All artists in their work, whether with the written word or with paint or dance or song, strive ultimately to seek resolution of problems and questions. This is what creating your journal, just like all art-making, can do for you.

That your bodily health can improve through writing about the past may seem at first hard to believe, until you remember what is now known about the power of your mind and emotional expression over your body. Other researchers besides Dr. Pennebaker have shown that writing like this has an immediate booster effect on your immunity. This in turn can come to your rescue whenever you're exposed to germs, and even more serious things like cancer-causing influences. People with as diverse and physical ailments as chronic asthma and rheumatoid arthritis have received significant symptom relief from these kinds of exercises, coupled of course with the best medical care.

Perhaps most vital is what regular journal and other forms of artistic writing can do for your general health and well-being. This is preventive medicine too—and it's certainly cost-effective. Whatever your life and health situation may be at the moment—whether you are a hospital patient or a family caregiver of someone with a serious illness, whether you are newly recovered from severe trauma or just coming to terms with long-term disability—writing regularly can be relied upon to help you. You'll sort out your ideas more easily, grasp new information more quickly, make big and daunting decisions more willingly. You'll also find yourself feeling more all-around creative in your life, as well as a lot happier in general. By no means least, you may notice significant improvements in your physical health.

Exercise: Feeling Words

Before saying a bit more about journaling, I'd like to give you one more easy exercise that will help you give voice to all your feelings, however deep they may be buried. There are hundreds and hundreds of words in the English language that describe different feelings, so it can be helpful to have a kind of *thesaurus* of them to refer to when you need it.

I'm going to give you a few commonly used words, and invite you to make a list for each that contains words with a similar meaning. The idea of this is to put yourself in touch with nuances of feeling. For example, "ecstatic" isn't quite the same as "excited." And "attentive" has a different sense from "curious."

These are the twelve words I have for you: happy, sad, unsure, overwhelmed, inspired, dull, joyful, desperate, grateful, restless, regretful, peaceful. Write down each of these words, and as you do so, brainstorm on each one for a couple of minutes, coming up with all the words that seem to have a similar meaning. Make your lists beneath each word in turn. This will probably take you about twenty minutes or so. When you've done this, take up your colored pencils, choosing a color you like and one you don't like. You're going to highlight, or underline, all the negative words—the *downers*—with your least favorite color, and highlight with your favorite color all the positive words, or *uppers*.

The last part of this exercise is to pick at random one downer word and one upper word. Make a sentence containing one of these words. Then start free-writing whatever comes into your mind. Keep going for five minutes, without pausing to think about it. When you've finished with this word, write a sentence containing the other word you chose, and free-write from there for another five minutes.

Tips for Authentic Journaling

Okay, now you've got yourself thoroughly loosened up for writing in your journal. I'm going to give you a few tips so you get the most out of it.

You've got—or should have—a lot of entries in your workbook by now. For the exercise you're going to do next, you may want to start a new book, rather than simply turning the pages of the old one. The reason is that from now on I'm going to urge you to journal regularly. I don't necessarily mean every day, even though the word *journal* is derived from the old French for "daily." I do suggest that you dedicate a book to this sole purpose, and keep your current workbook for everything else.

If you prefer to still use the same book for all your art entries, projects, and journaling, that's fine too. You may find you like your different kinds of art-making all mushed in together, keeping each other company, and perhaps feeding off each other. We haven't talked much about that yet, but being a *multimedia* artist rather than sticking to one medium is important for giving yourself the maximum benefit from making art. A hero of mine, William Carlos Williams, was not only for forty years a pediatrician with a busy single-handed practice in Rutherford, New Jersey, but is also called the father of modern American poetry. He penned his poems right alongside his clinical notes on his patients. What a marvelous example of the art of patient care side by side with the art of poem-making—all in the name of healing.

As far as starting to journal, always remember that whatever comes into your mind first is something that's been sitting right there in your memory banks just crying out to be noticed. It's sitting in wait, ready to flow out from your mind on to the paper, by means of your artist's pen or pencil. This is the way it can get *cleaned up*, like one of those messes we make every day on the kitchen counter or the bathroom floor. Only this one's been there for a while, patiently expectant. It's high time to deal with it, using this newfound art form of yours.

It's crucial to let yourself go and get right into your true thoughts and feelings about a given event or subject matter. Reflect for a moment and realize that all artists draw on their innermost selves, and often on their most raw and painful experiences. Do you know why? Because it's *healthy* to do so. It pulls those stored-up emotions out of you. That's the root purpose of all artistic expression. So start off thinking of yourself as the artist you are, drawing on your life experience as inspiration for your art. This is your story—this time of writing. No one else need share it, unless you choose for them to do so.

Beware of your mind's practiced skill at deflecting things at first too horrible to think about. Try hard not to do that. Stay with something that really hurt and wounded you at some time in your life, if that's what comes up first. It might be a tragic loss of a loved one, or something violent done to you when you were a child, once or repeatedly. It might be something you did or said that caused another a lot of hurt, and yourself shame and regret. It may have to do with something current or recent, linked with an illness or disability and its origins.

You should get into the habit of not searching too hard in your memories for a subject when you start to write. It will show itself to you if you just settle your body and mind, then wait and listen for a while. *First thoughts* are always the best guide to what's really going on. The trouble is that we get good at screening and filtering, so it takes practice to catch that first one, like a fish on your line. Almost subconsciously you'll lay it aside in favor of a second subject—a secondary one in significance to the real you but a bit easier to deal with.

Lastly, as with all the exercises in this book, it's helpful to repeat this one. You may find it easier and safer to work up to bigger traumas; it's just fine to stay with simpler stuff at first.

Exercise: Twelve-Speed Writing

Get yourself settled and take up your pen and paper—no computer word-processing for this exercise. You're going to be writing for fifteen minutes without pause. (Yes, without pause, so go to the bathroom first if you need to.) Most important, you're not going to worry one iota about grammar, spelling, or sentence structure. This is not the third grade and no one's looking over your shoulder with their pencil poised. This is just for you, if you hadn't grasped that yet. The main cause of writer's block is just that—the awful fear of judgment. Well, you're not going to be judged, not even by yourself.

Now for subject matter: You're going to take out of the closet something that's been sitting there, maybe for a while. I invite you to put down—without pausing or deflecting—your deepest feelings and thoughts about the worst, most upsetting experience you can dredge up from your memory banks, something that has affected you *profoundly*. Whatever presents itself to you right now is exactly what's on top of the pile, waiting to be taken out, looked at, and dealt with.

So let's go. Write first about the details of what happened, and then what you thought and felt about it at the time . . . all the details. Then write about how you feel about it *now*. How have your feelings changed? Does it still bother you as much now as at the time it first took place? Finally, write about how it might have been different, or what about the experience still needs to be resolved, and how you might do that. Don't start to analyze, though, until after you've finished your fifteen-minute block of free-flowing writing. Even then, avoid too much analysis. Stay with your feelings, and your intuition; go light on thinking and logic.

Don't worry if the tears come up. That's exactly what's supposed to happen, if you're still grieving about it. Some people end up with soggy pages and ink running, and that's just fine. The same with anger and even fear. You may have to shake some of this free. Odd, isn't it, that you should have fear about something long gone, but that's exactly what does happen. Unexpressed, these negative emotions get trapped within us, crusted over like unhealed internal wounds. It's high time to take up your pen and *let the stuff out*, as with a surgeon's scalpel on suppurating matter from an old wound.

Everyone has some such lesions. We could spend our lives uncovering little ones, but for this purpose I'm urging you to go for the gusto and address the more traumatic issues. Once again, no one's going to see this except you, unless you want them to. You can make it as illegible as you like, you can tear it up right after you write it, you can use invisible ink, or, as was popular in days gone by, you can keep your journal under lock and key. You can still buy those lock-up books for just that purpose in any stationery store.

Within your fifteen or twenty minutes, I want you to leave a couple of minutes at least to start taking a look at the issue in a *problem-solving, present-time way.* In other words, spend a little time reminding yourself of the obvious but often uncredited fact that this is *the past* you're writing about, that you're re-creating. This is a past that right now has absolutely no power over you—no power, that is, except any you may have been surrendering to it. It's like the way we revisit, sometimes endlessly, an old failed marriage, for example, with sadness or anger or resentment at our ex-spouse. This is simply giving your power away to the past: It's time to clean it up completely. You may have to return to it a few times, but I promise you that you can put this behind you for good. Just write some lines toward the end committing yourself to affirm your freedom from this bad memory. Also write about how you're going to make certain you never dwell on it again. Come back to these commitments as often as you need to.

Okay, you're done until the next time. Because I deliberately asked you to dig deep and come up with something pretty traumatic that happened to you, you may not feel too good right now. You may have managed to suppress this issue for many a year, and now you've opened it up again. So now you need to heal yourself and this issue fully and in a healthy way. You may well need to give yourself several sessions over the next two or three days or so, in order to work things out and complete the healing process. Or there may be someone you can trust to share all this with. It's just like after surgery or an accident—long-standing issues don't release their grip that quickly.

But they will, if you commit yourself to the task. The potential rewards for both your present-time and future health are immeasurable.

Poetry Therapy

There are many recent books about the benefits to your health of reading and writing poetry. Two of my favorites are those of licensed poetry therapist John Fox: *Poetic Medicine* (1997) and *Finding What You Didn't Lose* (1995). Both offer the simple prescription of poem-making for personal and collective healing. Poetry therapy has evolved over the past fifty years as a profession that uses poems and poem-making to help people deal with any manner of physical, emotional, and spiritual trauma. You can use all kinds of poems, your own or others', to put your often hard-to-express emotions into words. In so doing you'll add greatly to your self-understanding, your problem-solving ability, and your self-esteem.

Like everyone else, you can and do write poems, even if you've never acknowledged or even noticed it. The very act of putting words together in your mind and expressing them in your own voice to another person—*the best way you know how to make yourself understood and felt*—is a poetic act. Not that we always try very hard: much of what comes out of your mouth each day is of course repetitious, and not laden with much thought or emotion. Dr. Deepak Chopra says we have three hundred thoughts each day, two hundred and fifty of which we had yesterday. But there are many times each day when you do put conscious awareness and intuitive feeling into how you say things. As soon as you do that, you start to harness the inherent rhythm and beauty of words, in their couplets and chains and clusters. This is a natural human inclination, and words are a God-given gift, touching common ground between us.

In *Poetic Medicine* (1997, p. 3), John Fox sees poem-making as "a revelation, resurrection, and rebirth"—moments of freedom from limitation, in which you *surprise yourself* with your own and others' words of wisdom. Be it a cry or a sigh, a scream or a dream, a poem happens every time you express your authentic self without pretense or illusion. The more you practice this magical art, the further along your healing journey you'll travel.

Story: Fear

The woman on my phone at 2 A.M. sounded terrified. As well she might. Her twelve-year-old son, my patient, was dangerously ill with a high fever we couldn't explain. Earlier that night he'd had a prolonged epileptic seizure from which he'd recovered over an hour or two. We'd found no explanation for this complication either. And here was Julie, his mother, quite unable to sleep and desperate for explanation.

It isn't such an unusual thing even in modern medicine for doctors not to have all the answers. Medical students pack their four years of training with such a myriad of facts that many emerge thinking nothing can happen for which they won't have a rational explanation. Some think it's their sole task to dig deep enough with enough tests to uncover the cause and so cure the problem. Then they discover real life, where it doesn't always work out that way. Patients haven't read the textbooks and sometimes behave unpredictably.

I'd done everything I could that night in the way of tests, gotten his fever under control, and given him medicine to stop more seizures. I'd explained to his mom what was going on as best I could, and tried to calm the worst of her fears. Then I'd said a prayer and gone home to sleep, hoping she'd be able to do the same. It wasn't to be. Julie had stayed fully alert through the night beside his sleeping body, asking question after question of the darkness, of God, I guess: Why was all this happening to him, and to her? Where did she go wrong? What on earth could she do to help him? *Would he make it?*

Finally, exhausted and angry, she'd called me up with her pent-up questions. As she told me later, she realized she was feeling resentful that I could take off to my bed while she saw her son perhaps dying at any moment. Half awake, I felt the rush of her words coming over the line, demanding explanation for things we'd been over at length a few hours before. I didn't know what to say in the face of this outpouring, and I didn't have my thinking cap on straight anyway. So I just listened as she raged.

After a few minutes, both of us must have noticed the change in tenor of the conversation, even if we couldn't have acknowledged it. The rage was replaced first by tears, then by some rather rueful laughter on both our parts about the "craziness of kids, scaring us both like this." This is how she put it in the poem she wrote a day or so later about this incident—her first conscious poem in twenty years.

> I'm scared
> Why do they do this to a person?
> You bring em up to behave,
> say their prayers, wipe their noses,
> then they go and get sick
> and scare the willies out of you.
> The craziness of kids, scaring
> us both like this. He's doing his best,
> old doc, I guess he doesn't
> know it all after all.
> But I don't want him going to school
> on my son. God, stop scaring us

like this. And son, read the book
where it says, after the bit
about brushing your teeth
and not eating too much candy
and not staying out late, the bit about
not having fits—giving us fits.

The Instinct to Make Art

For me this is the therapy of poetry at its best. Julie wrote that poem some days after the event. She hadn't, she told me, written any poetry as an adult before this. I'm sure she was trying to capture what was niggling away in her mind, and so clean it up. Not to get rid of the event or the emotion attached to it, but simply to make it a happier and safer memory to recall. Poetry was the way to do it that came instinctively to her.

Whether she'd have written it if her son had died that night we'll never know. He didn't; but he remained very sick for weeks, and his mother had time to reflect on some pretty deep stuff. Why it came to her to put a poem on paper *at that time* we'll also never know. I can only remind you that we're all artistic beings, poets and painters and dancers and singers. Often the urge to create grabs you out of the blue at a critical moment. When it does, grab it right back. Don't ignore it. Your creator gave you this gift of divine inspiration for just such times as these. Stay tuned to those promptings when you're under stress; they can be your saving grace.

One thing about such apparently spontaneous impulses, though: They happen much more often to those who are already making a habit of art-making in their daily routine, however mundane it may feel. It's like the old saying: "Fortune favors the brave." If you're out there being brave (in this case in your attempts at making art) without letting the possible consequences deter you, then the light of saving fortune (in this case artistic inspiration) is more likely to smile on you.

Julie's poem is a mother's poem: simple but very elegant. It catches all sorts of things about how she was feeling, but mostly after she'd come through the first rush of fear, thinly disguised as anger. Perhaps she couldn't even remember the first part afterwards, because she'd been so crazy with fear. But she found a need to write something that almost chided her son for being the unpredictable boy he was, while still finding within herself the spontaneous courage of humor. By the end, the only anger she had left for me also came out humorously: "I don't want him going to school on my son."

This is above all a therapeutic poem for Julie. It takes a frightened mother's thoughts and feelings and puts them on paper in a short and potent way. What art!

Exercise: Putting Poetry to Work

Now it's your chance. This is your opportunity to put poetry to work for you. It's what poetry likes to do: make itself useful. You're going to write a poem just as though you'd never written one before. Perhaps you can't remember ever doing so. But I suspect we all put poems on paper as children—until we were scolded by our parents and teachers for wasting time, or laughed to shame by our friends.

Well, no one's going to laugh at you now. Because once more you'll be writing for an audience of one: yourself. If you choose to share your poem with others, that's hunky-dory. But start out with the assumption that you won't be doing so. You'll find it much more freeing. I'm not going to ask you to dredge up more horrors from your past life either—or your present one, even if there are any. This is an exercise in the art of poem-making, plain and simple, so the subject absolutely doesn't matter.

To get started, take a fresh page of your workbook and write down just three or four words on each of ten lines. Make it a fresh subject for each line. Just think about today's activities and chronicle them. If this is first thing in the morning, then cast your mind back over the events of yesterday. Or you can think over what is going to be happening today or tomorrow. What are a few memories or expectations? Thus . . .

Woke at seven

Stayed in bed till ten

Had a check-up with the doctor

Didn't eat my breakfast ("negative events" are fine too)

Called my sister

And so on, as mundane as that. Just jot down these short moments—*events*—that make up the sum of your day. But don't take long, just two or three minutes for these ten short items. And don't think too much; the everyday things are just fine for this purpose. You don't have to stretch yourself to recall momentous events. The point of this is to see for yourself how you can weave poems out of the plainest cloth.

Now put your book down, but hang onto your pen. Close your eyes and bring it down on the general area of the page where you've been writing. Which item has your pen picked out? That's the very one that's asking you to write a poem about it. If this feels too fanciful to you, well, poem-making is about indulging the fancifulness, the fantasies, within you.

I hope you've got it by now: You can write poems about anything. Indeed some of the best are written on the simplest topics, like the food on your table. You have the makings of ten poems right in front of you. The choice of topic is just a *way in.* It's important, but it's quickly passed over like any threshold as you enter into a whole new domain of creative possibility. Or, to use a different metaphor, you're going diving into the ocean of memory and fantasy opening up to you. If you're scared of getting out of your depth, don't know what monsters of the deep you're going to meet down there in your imagination, then just keep thinking of this whole thing as a game. Because that's what it is, just play. Play with good purpose, but play nevertheless.

Let's say you did indeed write the phrase "Stayed in bed till ten," and that your pencil landed on it. This would become the first line of the ten-line poem you're going to create. Pause for a moment, long enough to recall the time this line referred to: in this example, that time between waking up and getting up. As you start recalling the details of your own experience, start your hand moving your pencil across a fresh page. Keep the lines short, about the same length as the ones you've made already (three or four words). Put into those lines all you can remember of that time this morning or yesterday, for example, about your bed and you inside it: what you did, thought, decided, felt. It doesn't matter if you can't remember much. Use your intuition. Try this: If you *could* remember what thoughts and feelings you had, what would they be?

One very important thing: Don't think that the lines have to be complete in themselves, or grammatically correct, or that they must run on in sense and sequence one to the next, like you've been taught a prose sentence must do. Especially don't think the lines have to rhyme or scan (meaning have a set number of syllables each). This is free verse, okay?

Don't struggle with this, or with yourself. Relax. Let go of the need to get to the end, thinking that you've got to produce ten lines or you'll go to hell in a handcart. Just because I said you're to write ten lines, does that mean you have to? You're in charge. You can do exactly what you want, just like giving yourself permission to go beyond the margins of the circular mandala you made earlier. Such rule-breaking includes misspelling every single word if you want to. (That might make a pretty fine poem, actually.) This is play, remember? The time it takes for you to write this poem—it might be the first you've penned in half a century—is exactly how long it's supposed to take. Three minutes or thirty. It's just fine. If you need a nap in the middle, go for it.

Above all, don't worry about how *good* it is. Who's judging? Ah, you are? Well, have mercy on yourself. Love your frailty and uncertainty, right along with your artistry and creativity.

Your Unseen, Unseeing Audience

Okay, finish up now. Read back over what you've written. If you want to change anything, go right ahead. The first draft of a composition should be for fast and pure expression of whatever comes up in your memory and imagination. The next draft, if you choose to work on it, is for editing and polishing as you see fit. You can even rip the page out, crumple it up in a little ball, and toss it in the garbage.

But I hope you won't. Because I'd like you to read it *aloud* to me—your unseen and unseeing audience. Take your time with it. Poetry ever since prehistory was meant to be spoken or sung aloud. As I've said earlier, it was one of the earliest art forms put to the service of human healing, which was long before human beings had the means to write things down.

Notice as you read your poem aloud the rhythm of the words, of the lines. Listen to the sound of these words and phrases and sentences that you've ordered on paper in this unique way, about a piece of your very own life. Aren't they fine? Don't you love these little guys? They're here just for your service. And they're available in every shape and sort of sound, and combination of sounds. It's just like you used your newfound visual art skills to make colored doodles, simply to see how all the colors could mingle and match.

Words Are Workers

Count the number of different words you've used in this composition of yours. You have a personal vocabulary of several thousand, each one a worker on your behalf. The rhythm of your poem may be jerky or smooth, sluggish or staccato. That, just as much as the content, reflects the mood of the moments you've captured. It also reflects the mood of these more immediate moments during which you were building a lovely container on paper for these memories.

But what about the content? What came up for you—anything surprising? Who were you this morning, and now? Why did those things happen to you? Why did you do those things just then? How

much of it was thought through, and how much was quite spontaneous? How pleased are you with that short piece of your life, or how
disappointed, angry, sad? Where do all those feelings come from?
Where are you now, at this present moment, in your mind and spirit,
in relation to where you were then—the subject of your poem?

These are the kinds of questions creative writing tosses up.
Words are your prime communicator, both with others and with
yourself. Be thankful for them and use them freely. They're here to
attend to you, to help you be clearer in your thoughts, in expression
of your feelings. They're here to help you make up your mind about
things and about what to do next, and you can even use them to
predict what may happen in your life. They'll help you reclaim your
creative fire and passion, an ever-available medium for expressing
yourself with beauty and grace. There will always be beauty in whatever words you decide to use—even those of jealousy or hatred—
because they are speaking your version of the truth at that moment,
and because they are inherently beautiful in their form, rhythm, and
sound. Our creator made it that way. They're your servants, your
attendants—like angels.

6

Reclaiming Your Voice and Making Music

And finally, and perhaps best of all, we have music.

—Lewis Thomas

The Only Universal Tongue

This is how Victorian poet Samuel Rogers described the marvelous medium of communication we call music. Musical sound not only goes beyond differences in human speech, it even breaks down barriers between us and other species. Like many another pet owners, we often leave music playing for our two parrots to listen to when we're out all day. Not only will they imitate the sounds, but they'll often dance to the music too. As countless singers and songwriters have told us, there is music in the sound of the wind in the trees, the breaking of waves on the seashore, and the echo of far-off planes and trains. Music is the stuff of romance, of inspiration, of sacrament.

You may have read or heard about "the Mozart effect," the recent recognition of the potent effect that music of many kinds can have—to inspire, teach, and heal us from many ills. This is the term musicologist and sound healer Don Campbell captured in his 1997 book of the same name. Most of us grew up surrounded by music of all kinds, both the harmonies of nature and those contrived and created by humankind. It started with your mom, who sang you to sleep in your crib with lullabies. Actually, as we now realize, it started much earlier than that, with your first awareness of sound early in your second trimester *in utero* as you tuned into the rhythmic flow of placental blood, probably accompanied in time by your mother's cooings.

But it isn't only songs and symphonies that reach us in our innermost places of primal memory. The original meaning of the word *heal* comes from the Middle English to make *sound*, or whole, again. If you're one of the great majority born with intact hearing and vocal powers, you've been blessed with the ability to generate beautiful sounds. Pause and think about it. You use that ability for good every time you choose to speak gently or encouragingly, soothingly or lovingly, to another person.

Story: The Reader

When I was young, everyone had their tonsils out. It was a fashionable procedure for recurrent throat infections, done usually just before a child started school. (It's performed much less often nowadays.) I still recall having mine out at the age of six: a horrid experience. I was scared because no one told me what was going to happen when I got to the hospital. Or if they did, it didn't sink in. All I knew was that I felt physically fine and didn't know what the fuss was about. I never made any link between having the operation and the times the doctor had come to visit when I was laid up in bed with a temperature and a sore throat or earache. (Yes, they made house calls in those days.)

When I started to wake up from the anesthetic, I was dimly aware of an awful pain in the back of my throat and a desperate need to drink something. The nurse was annoyed when I whimpered hoarsely for water. I guess she knew what would happen, but finally she gave in and I promptly vomited up water and a great plug of something that looked live a bloody dead animal, although it was probably a temporary dressing to stop any bleeding I might have after the operation.

Then my mom was there, and things started looking up. In those days they didn't let parents into the wards much except on a strict schedule, so she wasn't allowed to be with me as I swam back into consciousness from the anesthetic. I was still hurting and nauseous, but it seems they couldn't give me more medicine by injection, and of course I couldn't swallow anything. But she had the answer, as always. She'd brought with her three of my favorite books: *Just So Stories*, *Wind in the Willows*, and of course *Winnie-the-Pooh*. Within minutes I'd entered that world of enchantment that the first words of those books could conjure up for me. They still can today.

"Here is Edward Bear, coming downstairs now, bump, bump, bump, on the back of his head, behind Christopher Robin. It is, as far as he knows, the only way of coming downstairs, but sometimes he feels that there really is another way, if only he could stop bumping for a moment and think of it. And then he feels that perhaps there isn't. . . ." (3). By this time my tears were forgotten, along with the pain and nausea, the strangeness and the fear. I was *gone*.

The Mirror of the Soul

The above story isn't for highlighting the story line, nor for recommending good reading matter for hospitalized people, although it does that too. What I want to do right now is remind you of something that I dearly hope you experienced many times as a child. That is, the rhythmic, monotonous, deeply soothing sounds of your favorite grown-up reading aloud to you. Because this is the ideal prescription, both for going to sleep for your operation and for waking up from it. Only lullabies are closer to womb sounds. Nursery rhymes certainly ought to resemble lullabies, although for some inexplicable reason they are mostly frightening little morality tales, at least in my English tradition.

The ideal thing for you when you're really in need of comfort is to have a book read to you that is so familiar you could finish every sentence before the words are spoken. It's the *familiarity* that's so essential a part of the healing ritual, like favorite hymns in church if you're a Christian. Although I'm now a Quaker and we worship in silence, I'm still deeply moved by the music of the Anglican tradition that raised me. I'm sure this is the case for every other form of worship. The moments of receiving this *communion* from one for whom you have the deepest trust and love are profoundly sacred. This is the music of the spheres.

Healing Sound

This chapter is about sound and healing. I'll mostly be talking about sounds made by humans, although not exclusively. Much healing sound is taken from nature, and it's now blessedly available via audiotapes and CDs. The sounds of the sea, wind, rain, birds, and whales and other animals can extend an awesome but totally safe power over you. They touch things deeply primal. You can readily be hypnotized by their endlessly repeated rhythms and uplifted to a transcendent realm of safety. In these moments of listening, you are surely with your maker. I believe that if you listen well enough, you will get answers to all life's questions. I'm speaking of those profound questions like "Who am I?", "Why am I here?", "Where am I going?", "Why is this happening to me?", and "What should I do?"

Exercise: Bedtime Reading

This exercise will help you get in touch with the subconscious underpinnings of your aware and waking life. All you'll need is a favorite book from your childhood. You may well have to get a copy from the library or bookstore; if so, you'll find it in the children's section, of course. I've already mentioned a few of my favorites: English books because I started life in England. You may well turn to *Charlotte's Web* or *The Little Prince* or *Stuart Little*. It's best for this exercise if you have a very close friend or family member beside you, but it's not essential. You can be your own mom (that goes for you men too) and do this for yourself.

Whether you're alone or have your friend to minister to all your needs, get yourself settled in your comfiest spot. In bed is best, because it's nice and warm and cozy. Make certain you're not going to be disturbed for half an hour or so. Get the lighting *just so*. Puff up your pillows, and nestle under the covers with just your head and arms free. If you're not alone, you can tuck your arms in too, because what you're doing is recreating a kind of *womb*. Just wriggle about until you're quite certain you could never in a thousand years be more comfy and content.

Open your book at the very beginning or have your companion do so. All the best stories start at the beginning, long long years ago, with "Once upon a time ..." Now here are the instructions for the reader—yourself or your companion: Start reading *aloud*. Begin quietly, unhurriedly, soothingly. Let your voice pick up the rhythm and cadence of the words. Listen. Listen to the words flow, like the waves of the sea, the tumble or trickle of water along the river's bank, the monotonous, soothing sound of rain beating on the roof of your home long ago. Let your eyes drift across the page, and your voice with it. Keep your breathing slow and deep, your voice even and quiet. Just keep going until your companion is asleep. Or until your book drops from your grasp as you drift away to dreams of forests and mountains and seasides and days of endless sunshine. . . .

Making Yourself Heard

Ah! What a nice experience. You know you can come back to this whenever you need to make a mind-trip and get away for a while. Store it up, this well-kept secret. All these stories of childhood are there just waiting for you to reclaim them. You only need your very favorites, and you'll never get bored with this ritual. Have you noticed how young children want the very same story or will watch the same video over and over again? I know some who've fallen asleep to *Cinderella* or *Beauty and the Beast* well over a hundred times while in a hospital bed.

The human voice is the simplest form of music therapy I know. For be in no doubt, it *is* music. It is breath, vibration, the divine spirit of inspiration and expiration. It is with us from the baby's first cry, and its answering maternal coo, to everyone's last dying utterance on this earth. Your voice is a remarkable healing instrument, "the mirror of the soul," as the Roman orator Publius Syrus called it. It has immeasurable power to heal. Music can enlarge your horizons, bring you peace and harmony, connect and center you, offer you nurturance and protection. So now's your chance to reclaim this universal force. You've been silent too long, and deaf to its joyful energies. Your own vocal artist is at your service, as it has always been.

Story: A Hummer

There's a man I'll call Drew whom I knew for a while. I haven't seen him in a year or two, but I know he's fine. He couldn't but be fine, given his lust for life, which emanated from him.

How I know this was from his singing. This was something it seems he did all the time. He was always quiet about it though—as though he respected silence, and the need of others to have this precious commodity around them sometimes. But come close enough to him, and you'd notice he was always singing. Often I'd pick up the hum from a few feet away, when he was in bed in his striped pajamas and I dropped by to visit for a while. I never recognized any tunes among the assortment of notes that came softly billowing forth, but it was music just the same.

To sit there beside him brought forth in me an extraordinary memory. I would always recall myself as a boy of eight lying in the sun outside the entrance to Cheddar Gorge, the network of underground caves in the Cheviot Hills in Somerset, which is the English county where I was raised. I'd often lie there listening to the distant, harmonious echoes of people touring the inside of the caves to see the stalagmites and stalactites. That's what Drew's singing sounded like—echoes of something deep within. It was very calming, very spiritual. Such is music's ability to carry you instantly back in your mind-travels to your early beginnings.

Drew was in his late seventies when I knew him. He'd had circulation problems for many years, and in recent times had developed nasty leg ulcers that didn't heal well. He lived alone by choice, an independent, some might say stubborn old man. He had pretty limited resources, and the region where he lived was poorly served by home health care agencies. He just couldn't do what he really needed to do to get his legs patched up, which was to elevate them to bring the swelling down and let them rest and mend. He couldn't manage the cleaning and dressing of his lower legs easily either, and the ulcers would often get infected, forcing him into the veteran's administration (VA) hospital for several spells. One of our artists met him during a visit and told me about his song-humming habits.

I never heard him sing a song out loud in the times I met him. I asked him once about this habit of his. It was obvious he was hardly aware of it, it was so ingrained. He thought about it for a while, then said: "I s'pose it helps me concentrate when I get a bit unclear about things. And it keeps me happy, you know. Whenever I'm a bit out of sorts I just start up humming and I feel better." For all his limitations and his frailty, Drew was one of the happiest souls around. He gave off a spirit of happiness and repose without having to declare it.

Actually he never said much, and after my first visit, when it was obvious he didn't want to talk a lot, I took to visiting him for a bit of peace and quiet myself. "Talking tires me," he said once, but I never worked out if he meant physically or mentally. He said he liked me coming to see him though, so I'd just sit and listen to his music. His tunes were very melodious, like harmonies, varying in pitch and rhythm quite a bit. They were lovely, and it was peaceful to be around him.

Why Sing?

So that's music and healing for you. I like to ask the questions: Why does the bird sing? Is it because it wants to show how happy it is or is it in order for it to feel happier, less lonely or scared? My answer is assuredly the latter. It's like laughing in the dark wood to cheer yourself up. I think Drew developed the habit of singing to himself—and to anyone else who happened into range—not just to lift his spirits but to maintain them at their always happy level, whatever was happening. So I want to explore this phenomenon of musical sound with you and offer you some tips on how to make it work for you.

Music therapy has been around for as long as we have, although we didn't always call it that. Have you ever whistled in the dark? Sung to your baby to settle him to sleep? Joined in the ritual of the local team's chant to rouse them to victory? Sung in church or synagogue or mosque or whatever religious institution you were raised in? These are timeless rites of human expression, giving voice to joy and sorrow, fear and sacred praise.

The first musical instrument was of course the human voice, each one in some ways imitative of every other, yet possessed of its own unique qualities. "I'd know that voice anywhere." Absolutely right: there's never been, nor ever will be, two exactly the same. Your voice carries your character, personality, mood, intelligence, your very genetic makeup contained within its dulcet tones. And every musical instrument that's ever been developed carries some of the qualities of our voices. That's what's so appealing about them.

If you can speak, you can sing, as someone nicely said. And even if you're without a larynx (a voice box) and haven't yet learned to use your esophagus (your gullet) to make meaningful sounds, you can still *give voice*. You can still sing silently and hear the notes inside your mind. That's what the imagination is for. Look at Beethoven, who while stone deaf could still compose in his mind transcendently beautiful symphonies. What after all is singing but varying the pitch and cadence and rhythm of your voice a little more in order to make art? Yes, we're back to art-making, define it how you will. I'm talking about taking sound, which can be an ugly, cacophonous thing when distorted and intensified, and molding it in your mind and larynx, or on any musical instrument you want, to make lovely melodies.

This urge to give voice in song is a human rite, and a right, we all possess. It's your right to *sound* (to use a verb that's getting popular nowadays). Sound is simply energy you can organize into any combination of patterns and shapes, frequencies and intensities, traveling in waves of vibration between and around us. It's the sound of the human voice that has generated all the genres that have been born of this vocal music-making: from choral chants to ragtime, from chamber and cathedral music to rap and rock and roll. It's primarily, primally, about harmonizing, chiming, blending, synchronizing, syncopating, rejoicing. Because our souls are driven to do so, and they'll suffer in silence when suppressed. The essayist Thomas Carlyle called music "the speech of angels." It's no accident that we've adopted into our language phrases like striking a familiar chord, being in harmony, or on the same wavelength, with others, feeling out of sync, and getting a tune-up.

Exercise: Sounding

Let's try another easy exercise (and it's all easy). If you can, stand up straight, or if you're in bed, sit up as straight as you can, preferably with your legs dangling over the side. Take two or three deep breaths, as deep as you can. It may set you off coughing, if you're not used to really expanding your lungs. If so, get yourself a glass of water and start over. I know I've urged you to breathe deeply a few times before many of the exercises you've done already, to get in a relaxed and receptive frame of mind. But now you're really going to focus particularly on your breathing pattern, in order to get yourself well prepared for the art of sounding.

See if you can breathe deeply without moving your shoulders up and down. This is diaphragmatic breathing, or breathing from your belly. Watch the movement in and out of your abdomen. It should be expanding outward as you breathe in, and vice versa, like babies' bellies do. It may take some practice if you've gotten out of the habit of using mainly your diaphragm for breathing, as many of us have. If your shoulders are rising up to meet your ears, this means you're using mostly your chest and neck muscles, which are accessory, not primary, muscles of breathing. Keep practicing until you see that mighty diaphragmatic muscle moving your belly in and out below your ribs.

Now as you get into the swing of this, into the conscious rhythm of deep breathing, start making some sounds on the out-breath—just like audible sighs. Don't think about what sounds yet; just let them come. Enjoy playing with making noises like babies experiment with sounds. Try a groan, or a sigh, or an expression of anticipation or joy.

Now try a few vowels more consciously: AY-EE-I-O-YU-AH-OO-UH and so on. Draw out the sounds a bit. Then stretch them even longer, just sighing them out. Drink some more water if you need to, to lubricate your larynx and loosen things up. Play with these different sounds, just as if you'd never heard them before. Keep consciously relaxing, not forcing anything. Now try putting a bit of expression in. Try a wail of anguish first. Then offer a cry of joy. Try an exclamation of surprise, then a shouted gesticulation of pain, then a mighty guffaw of laughter.

Now let's try making some music with these sounds. This simply means you put a little more melody and harmony, a bit more expression and feeling into it. Just a little is fine—there's no rush with this. Finally, try joining the sounds together in a chain, which you'll soon find amounts to a little song, or at least a Winnie-the-Pooh hum. Try a sad song. Then put out a happy one. How about a song of triumph? Then offer your audience, seen or unseen, a romantic ballad or a jazz tune. Pick up the tempo a bit and start rocking. Ha, there you go, tapping your feet to the beat.

Robbed of Our Birthrights

How many of us have been cut off from this inherent right to sound off and let our voices be heard? How many of us were told as school-children to "just mouth the words," or that we "couldn't carry a note"? I have my own version of this. Whenever as a young teenager I would burst into song, my aunt who raised me would at once ask: "Where does it hurt most?" This comment soon shut me up from ever singing at home, even though the school choirmaster saw fit to let me sing baritone in the choir. Woody Guthrie, on the other hand, had encouraging words for everyone. He said that as far as he was concerned, harmonizing was singing any note no one else was singing at the time.

So, if you can speak you can sing. And if you can move you can dance. (But that's another story, one for the next chapter.) Your first task right now is to forget any messages you've received at any time in your life that you're a tuneless, humless, rhythmless clod. If you're alive you've got rhythm, baby.

Story: The Proof of the Pudding

I'm borrowing this story—much shortened—from sound healer Don Campbell's best-selling book *The Mozart Effect* (1997, p. 7), which probably has the most up-to-date and comprehensive review of the scientific research on music and health. Many other people have written about music being used to improve your overall health and well-being. Other books that are very worthwhile for a layperson to read are Hal Lingerman's *The Healing Energies of Music* (1995) and Laeh Maggie Garfield's *Sound Medicine* (1987).

Don tells the extraordinary but entirely believable tale of how he rid himself in three weeks of a blood clot lodged deep in his brain. All he did was hum to it, and while doing so hold a constant image of its resolution. He'd been getting terrible headaches, seeing flashes of light in front of his eyes, and seemed to be losing his vision. He experienced his humming as having "warmth, brightness, and clarity . . . a vibrating hand coming into my skull on the right side, simply holding the energy within." He would offer up a vowel sound traveling throughout his body for about three minutes, as his breathing slowed and he felt calm and fully present in his body.

He knew he had to hum without too much power, to make sure he didn't break the clot off, just like a soprano can shatter a glass by holding a particularly high note. Sure enough, after three weeks of quiet humming and visualizing, the medical tests were repeated and showed almost complete resolution of the potentially lethal clot in his brain. It had shrunk from an inch and a half to one eighth of an inch.

Music has been used in all kinds of health care settings, from obstetrics to hospice programs. These are some of the things that melodies of different kinds can do in different settings: relieve your anxiety, ease your awareness of pain, inspire you to greater physical effort, clarify your thinking so you perform mental tasks better, and evoke your deepest spiritual responses. Some of the ways people in the hospital have been shown to benefit include faster recoveries after surgeries, strokes, and heart attacks; less anxiety and higher tolerance during painful treatments such as injections and dental care; and less nausea among patients with cancer receiving chemotherapy. People with long-term illness, and those who are facing the end of their lives, have been especially helped by building music into their hospital and home environments (Standley 1991).

Story: Getting a Head Start

Katie, a senior medical student friend of mine, came to see me one day last year to discuss what she'd been reading about music being introduced into newborn nurseries. We now know that the unborn baby is listening all the time, especially to the continuous rhythm of the placental *drumming* of its mother's heartbeat. Everyone has had the experience of being lulled to sleep by rhythmic sounds, like the tick of a clock or the waves of the sea, that reproduce this elemental musical link. We know that unborn babies even show their likes and dislikes to different types of music. When uterine sounds are combined with women singing lullabies, and played to newborns on a regular basis, they will be less agitated and more alert, and will grow and develop more quickly. Similar soothing music has been extended to premature and very sick babies, with excellent results in terms of increased weight gain and shorter hospital stays (Kaminski 1996).

Katie had read that the governor of Georgia had passed into law an act mandating that all nurseries have appropriate music available for newborn babies to hear, and had assigned the funds to pay for the program statewide. An Atlanta company aptly named Placenta Music had produced a series of cassette tapes of lullabies, which they mingled with the rhythmic sound of the blood pulsing between mother and baby in the womb. They had chosen this combination of sounds and rhythms on the basis of what is known to soothe, invigorate, and *attune* babies to their surroundings. This doctor-to-be wanted to do the same thing in our hospital. The newborn nursery already had a small supply of cassette tapes, but they weren't getting played regularly because the staff didn't have the time to devote to it. So we planned to have the students work out a rotation to go into the nursery two or three times a day and play the tapes.

But we ran into more difficulties than we'd anticipated in getting the program up and running, because of fears by staff members that the students wouldn't follow the strict protocols of the newborn nursery, where many sick babies are nursed on artificial ventilators and other life-supporting equipment. Katie and her buddies had to jump through many hoops and talk to several committees before getting permission to go forward. Even then they were restricted to babies in the least intensive section of the neonatal unit. But finally came the day when the students, armed with their own collection of tapes of lullabies and womb sounds, could go and meet the chosen newborns and their parents. Now every breakfast, lunch, and after-school time finds a bunch of these young healers moving from crib to crib switching on the lullaby tapes connected to speakers under the babies' pillows.

Who benefits from all this? The babies for sure—the research tells us so. And the parents too get to see this extra attention being paid to their newborn offspring, with healing intent. The staff certainly benefit, because this musical environment in which their charges are being cared for heightens their awareness of the importance of art married to science in medicine. Not least, these doctors-to-be themselves reap the reward of a chance early in their careers to learn how they can nurture the sick in the most loving and artful way possible.

Exercise: Sound and Noise

This is a two-part exercise that will familiarize you with the vital distinction between *sound* and *noise*. I hope it will give you some pointers for how you can take a stand against noise pollution, especially in hospitals. A hundred years ago, Robert Koch, a scientist who contributed a lot to our understanding of the spread of infection, predicted that we'd one day have to combat noise the way we once combated cholera and the plague. He was right. Noise pollution has become an epidemic hazard of modern life.

So take up your workbook. Divide the page with a vertical line into left and right columns. On the left you're going to make a list of ten sounds you consider harmonious. Obvious and universal ones are most birdsong, a mother's voice to her newborn, the waves of the sea, and so on. It won't take you long to come up with your ten. Now on the other side of the page make a list of ten sounds you find discordant or irritating. I think at once of a jackhammer pounding a hole in the road outside, a man and a woman screaming at each other in the next apartment, strident rock music coming from a car that pulls up beside you with its windows open, or the frequent overhead speaker on a hospital's paging system. See what you can come up with.

Now think some more about the hospital environment. This will be pretty easy if you frequent a hospital clinic or inpatient unit. Start another page, again with two columns but without any set length to your lists. Just think about, or—if you're there now—become aware of all the sounds you can hear, and assign them to one column or the other. For instance, voices—are they mostly harmonious or discordant? Add a few words of description if you've put the human voice in both columns. What about machines? At first thought you might think they're all annoying, but maybe that isn't so. What about the TV—how are the sounds on it predominantly? Calming, uplifting, or a cacophony? Some people fall asleep to the sound of the TV, so perhaps its noise isn't always that bad. Personally I prefer music without pictures, the sort of soothing meditative sounds that are often used by massage therapists or yoga teachers to add to the calming environment.

So what have you got, on the credit side and on the debit side? Did you think about the combination of the telephones, the computers, the pagers going off, the overhead announcements—often simultaneously—that merges into raucous turbulence?

Exercise: Combating Noise Pollution

Now for the second part of this exercise. I don't know anyone yet who's come up with more *positive* than *negative* sounds in a hospital environment. But I have every expectation you'll see such a state of grace in your lifetime. I believe we'll all come to recognize that a hospital should be like one big birthing room. The 150-odd birthing rooms scattered throughout the health care systems of our country are places where a mother can give birth in a homelike atmosphere, supported by her family and friends, where the sights, smells, and sounds are friendly, comforting, and healing. You don't meet the kind of resistance there that the medical students encountered in our newborn nursery. I see clear signs that these sweeping and necessary changes will be made—are starting to be made—in our places of health care.

Meanwhile, remember what I wrote in chapter 3 about creating a sacred place for your creative efforts. I stressed your need to *know* that you can take charge of your surroundings, even if you have to be seen as what is sometimes called "a difficult patient" in order to accomplish this. So now is your chance to do just this with ambient sound. How can you eliminate, or at least lessen, all the discordant sounds around you? How can you augment the harmonious, soothing, invigorating sounds whenever you choose to? What about getting rid of all sound when you want? Can you do that and still function? Ever tried those foam earplugs for airplane trips? They work like a dream. Ear plugs and a sleep mask are at the top of my list when I have to pack a bag for an airplane journey or a hospital stay. Isn't it ironic that face masks are so commonplace in hospitals, but simple equipment to shield eyes and ears is rare?

So look over your list and see what items in your negative column you can eliminate, and what in your positive column you can enhance. Now you need to set about taking the necessary steps or having a friend or family member do so. It may take a while (and some planning) to work out a routine, even a relocation, that allows you to be free of televised noise, for example. You may have to make repeated requests to have your door closed against external sounds. If you're in for a long hospital stay, you may want to arrange for drapes and other temporary furnishings to muffle sounds around you. White noise generators have rightly become popular recently for eliminating noisy surroundings and helping you be calmer, if your pocketbook allows it.

Now on the positive side, I'm sure you've included music, hopefully in many forms, for various moods and situations. You'll want different cassettes tapes or CDs for settling yourself down the night before surgery from the ones you'll use to get you going, rocking and rolling out of bed and into the bathroom a couple of days later. If you know you're going to the hospital, take yourself and your spouse or best friend to the store to stock up on some new music. Or you may well have a neglected collection at home that will fit every purpose, from helping you focus when you have difficult decisions to make to letting your emotions free when you're feeling sad or scared.

And don't forget some fun stuff in the form of children's songs, which are irresistible for cheering up folks of all ages. Try MCA's *Singable Songs for the Very Young*, by Raffi, or Warner Brothers' *In Harmony* by the Sesame Street Gang. Get down! And of course there are endless New Age recordings that are used as an adjunct for imagery and meditation purposes. I've found some of the best titles in the more alternative bookstores and even health food stores. One of the best resource organizations offering hope and inspiration to hospitalized people through music and the arts is Hospital Audiences, Inc. (See References.)

Different Strokes for Different Folks

Worldwide there are literally thousands of musical genres. Many are especially designed to express a particular sense or emotion. A few examples from our own culture are church hymns and chants, which give voice to the sacred in its many forms; jazz songs, which arose out of the laments of Southern black people's oppression as slaves; country-and-western songs, which originated with white European settlers in the South, and often serve to bemoan a love affair gone awry; folk music, which carries down traditions among a particular culture from generation to generation; and big-band music, which gets you dancing and romancing joyfully.

Many pieces of great music will uplift you in body, mind, and spirit. But of course we all have different tastes in the sort of compositions we enjoy, be they classical, country and western, jazz, or rock and roll. Music of different tempos and rhythms, and played on different instruments, will also have varying effects on you. The research studies tell us that once you get acquainted with its effects, you can use music both to energize you to dance or simply get out of bed and to relax you and soothe you to sleep. Some music will especially get to your emotions and have you crying or smiling freely. Other music, most of all that used in churches and synagogues, seems to speak directly to your spiritual self.

You may be a fan of Beethoven and Bach, of Willie Nelson and Dolly Parton, of Barbra Streisand or Miles Davis. Whatever your preference, it's well worth your while to take a look at what kind of music suits you in different situations and identify what it is about individual sounds and tempos and rhythms that especially appeals to you. For example, most people find that percussion instruments, from drums to brass bands, are arousing to the body, while stringed instruments, such as violin or guitar music, tend to have more emotional effects on us. The organ and the harp are often more soulful and will help you make a connection with deep feelings of divinity within you. Hal Lingerman's *The Healing Energies of Music* has some very detailed lists of music for all moods and occasions, although it's mostly limited to the classical composers. Even if you've never listened to a symphony or a piano concerto in your life, this might be something you want to explore. It can open up a whole world of experience that you might never have known about. Some examples of more well-known music include the marches of Mozart and Beethoven for energizing your physical body, Brahms' Hungarian Dances or Chopin's waltzes to get you up on your feet and dancing, some of the piano concertos of Beethoven, Tchaikovsky, or Rachmaninoff for relieving feelings of fear or grief, numerous woodwind pieces by Vivaldi and Ravel for relaxation and visualization, and Bach's Brandenburg Concertos to clear your head and get you thinking straight. If you do settle down to explore your tastes in music more deliberately, it will help to take notes in your workbook as you listen without other distraction to different pieces, and note their effects on your mood and thoughts.

Exercise: Musical Memories

Few of us can imagine a world without music. Music serves to soothe and relax you, arouse and inspire you, create a sacred presence, or simply get your feet tapping. If you or a loved one are ill, it's important to have a library of different musical sounds that will serve these many purposes whenever you need them. This is an exercise in recalling all the music that has appealed to you over the years, and then going about putting it all together in a handy collection.

Before you start recalling any music you'd like to have accessible, you need to be in a receptive mode. So get comfortable and make sure you're not going to be disturbed for a while. It may be helpful if you can darken the room. You certainly need to minimize external noise like TV and other distractions. Outdoor noises are mostly fine though, and if you can be outside where there are sounds of birds or wind or running water, then they will merge perfectly with your vocal memories. Now start to breathe deeply, and let your body and mind relax.

Cast your mind back to the earliest memories you have of hearing music. You may not recall your mother singing to you as an infant, although some lullabies may come to mind. You may recapture children's voices in a school choir or a congregation singing in a church when you were a young one. What about early nursery rhymes or other simple songs you had to learn? I remember singing "Row, row, row your boat" and "Way down upon the Suwannee river" when I was about five years old. They still stir memories when I hear them. After a few minutes, move on to your early memories of love songs or other popular songs on the radio or on records. What about more recently? What music have you heard in recent years that has appealed—soothed or stirred or inspired you? Are there tunes or melodies you find running through your head that would be good to have available whenever you wanted? You might have heard an especially uplifting musical score at a movie. These are almost always available on cassette tape or CD.

I mentioned a few classical music composers above, and you may already have a liking for the classics. If you haven't I strongly recommend you give it a try. Although modern popular music can certainly give pleasure, there's good reason why classical music stands the test of time. Here's a list of some of my favorite composers and their compositions, most of which are recommended as particularly therapeutic pieces of music: Bach's *Jesu Joy of Man's Desiring, Sheep May Safely Graze, Christmas Music,* and *Toccata and Fugue in D;* Beethoven's *Pastorale (no. 6) Symphony* and *Emperor Piano Concerto,* Brahms' *Lullaby* and *Piano Concertos;* Chopin's *Nocturnes;* Copland's *Appalachian Spring;* Debussy's *Afternoon of a Faun* and *Claire de Lune;* Dvorak's *New World Symphony (no. 9);* Gershwin's *Rhapsody in Blue;* Grieg's *Piano Concerto in A;* Handel's *Water Music;* Haydn's *Creation* and *Toy Symphony;* Holst's *The Planets;* Mendelssohn's *Violin Concerto;* Mozart's *symphonies no. 39, 40 and 41 (Jupiter), Horn Concertos,* and *A Little Night Music;* Prokofiev's *Peter and the Wolf;* Pachelbel's *Canon in D;* Rimsky-Korsakov's *Scherherazade;* Schubert's *Ave Maria* and *Unfinished Symphony;* Tchaikovsky's *1812 Overture, Romeo and Juliet,* and *Swan Lake;* Vivaldi's *The Four Seasons;* Vaughan Williams' *Fantasia on a Theme of Thomas Tallis;* Paul Winter's *Earthbeat* and *Whales Alive;* and Zamfir's *Music for Flute of Pan.*

Many hospitals and almost all public libraries have collections of cassette tapes or CDs, so it shouldn't cost you anything to sample some of these pieces. You'll find something to suit every mood, from sacred and inspirational to children's and seasonal music, music for calm and meditation, music for concentration and focus, music to get you moving and shaking. I promise you it will be well worth your investment of time—and perhaps modest funds—to put together a collection of a couple of dozen tapes or CDs.

Exercise: Singing a Funny Song

You'll need at least one companion for this one. It should be someone you trust or who's shared in other art-making activities with you. You're going to sing like you've probably never sung before. That goes without saying, actually, because no matter how often any of us sings a song it will be a unique rendition each time, with a personality all its own.

Are you nervous about singing? Maybe you're hearing all those messages that told you "No way!" Well, here's your salvation, out from those traps of personal music-funks and low sing-self-esteem. You're going to take your courage from that story of impromptu

Thanksgiving singing that introduced this book to you, and all that it stands for. Remember the message: Art-making is a joyful, inspiring, and *safe* activity that will do you a world of good. You just have to get those support people together, remind yourself once more that you're an artist—meaning a painter, a poet, a clown, a dancer, *and* a singer—and then *let go and let God.*

Here are the words of the song I've chosen for you. I deliberately picked a funny one so you and your audience of supporters would spend so much time laughing you wouldn't have time to be nervous. Remember that your companions won't be laughing *at* you, only *with* you. They'll be thinking what a fool they would make of themselves if they tried it, and that that would be just fine. It may help you to remember that in medieval times the jester or *fool* was the only one who could get away with just about anything without kindling the king's wrath—and was often one of the few to survive at court.

Here goes:

I want to be a friend of yours,
Mmm, and a little bit more!
I want to be a pal of yours,
Mmm, and a little bit more!
I want to be a little flower
Growing at your door.
I want to be your . . .
Grandfather, grandmother,
Father, mother, sister, brother,
Mmm, and a little bit more—hey!

The point of this song is to practice it until you can sing it very quickly. Try saying it through a few times first, to get your tongue around those last three lines. Speak the lines slowly at first, then gradually speed up. Now start clapping to the beat that you're automatically creating, until you've got a rhythm down. Then get your audience to join in with the clapping and tapping of their toes until you're all jamming together.

But you're the one who's going to do the singing. They can join in in a few minutes, once you've shown them how—and you can all keep a straight face for long enough. If you don't know the song, or the tune, you can just make it up, but try singing it to the rhythm you've created. All you have to do is switch very gradually from a speaking to a singing voice. Play around with it until you're singing the whole thing. Try it slowly at first then gradually pick up the beat, or the speed. Okay, once you've shown them how to do it, they can join in too. Fluff the words and the notes as often as you like: Just keep going, all of you together. Keep telling each other that harmonizing is simply singing any note no one else is singing—remember? Now try to listen to yourself as you sing along. How does it sound? Sing up if you can't hear yourself over the others. You're the soloist, remember?

Practice Makes Perfect

Singing songs is something we all need to do more often. It's the most powerful way we have of giving voice to all our joys and sorrows, and there's good reason why dozens and dozens of different types of song-making and music-making exist, just in our culture alone. Music has been found to increase milk production by cows, slow traffic in city streets, enhance the quality of the traditional Japanese wine called *sake*, and speed up the learning of English by new immigrants.

So now that you've oiled your perhaps rusty vocal cords, set yourself a commitment to begin each day with a song. Get yourself a songbook of the sort of songs you're familiar with, so you don't have to learn unfamiliar tunes or words. Sing-songs are another thing I predict will become part of the regular scene in our hospitals and other places of healing. Indeed, there are already weekly sing-songs in our hospital's bone marrow unit that draw out many folks who are often very ill, to listen and—with a little encouragement—join in.

7

Performing Your Part

I'm scared all the time! I just act as if I'm not.

—Katherine Hepburn

Your Roles in Health and Illness

So far we've taken a close look at the visual, language, and musical arts as resources when you or someone close to you is ill. These are all for the most part static art forms; that is, I haven't asked you to move your body too much. In the next two chapters I'm going to introduce you to some forms of art-making that will involve you in more movement, or performance, of various kinds. Perhaps I've left these specific activities until last because they do ask a little more of you. They ask you to break away a bit from most adults' accustomed ways of being. But if you've stayed with me so far, you're well warmed up for what's to come.

"All the world's a stage, and all the men and women merely players . . ." wrote William Shakespeare. The theater, of all art forms, offers a metaphor for life in all its ups and downs, its episodes of tragedy and comedy. This is why it's such a particularly good resource for helping you get in touch with issues and problems that may be besetting you today. The field of drama therapy has long been used to unite the art of theater with the science of psychotherapy. It's a marvelous aid for restoring vitality and spontaneous feelings. Too often these have become stifled and suppressed by the troubles and traumas of everyday life. But you don't have to have a psychological illness to benefit from the therapy of drama and dance. Such techniques are commonly used in rehabilitation and senior citizens' centers, professional training and continuing education programs.

Hospitals are starkly concrete and *immediate* places, bringing those who find themselves there as patients (and their families) face-to-face with life's uncompromising realities. In the way that real-life dramas are played out against a background of emergency or operating rooms, waiting areas or intensive care units, hospitals provide a kind of continuous live theater, with everyone involved either as actors or audience. Because drama doesn't often happen in isolation; it's almost always an example—a depiction—of human interaction. The word *drama* comes from the Greek word meaning simply "doing things" or "action." It's on a par with the word *poetry*, which means simply "making things." Through drama, people explore ways to communicate verbally, physically, and emotionally. So if you find yourself in such a setting, on the receiving end of illness and its treatment, it can be enormously helpful for you to deliberately cultivate these skills. They will help you in your day-to-day interactions with everyone with whom you come in contact.

Story: Tracy on Stage

Four o'clock in the afternoon: a low time of day. Sid's back in the basement, hanging out with his new acquaintances, hardly what you'd call friends. Not yet; everyone's defenses are up.

This windowless space serves as home for a bunch of depressed teenage diabetics who refuse to take their shots. You might almost say they've decided that a life lived with diabetes isn't worth the paper it's printed on—only they don't have a choice. They've just left school for the day, where they've had the chance to mix again with their healthy peers. But the barrier of chronic incurable illness seems to separate them, even from each other. So here they are, sitting around waiting for their next enforced shot, stuck in their own thoughts.

Sid's here for his weekly session, only he's not a patient. He's a professor of theater and literature at the university, here to do acting exercises with the teenagers. Sid always relished what poet Robert

Frost called "the fascination of the difficult." He's used to the safety of the comfy Saturday-night middle-class audiences he and his students draw to the university's Constans Theatre: faculty couples, appreciative fellow students, the local community. But he's not daunted by the thick silence surrounding him in this dismal space. He's toured the state's prisons, so he knows all about winning over "dead audiences." He's going to stretch this lot and their diaphragms, no matter what.

There's only one girl among the group of six. Fifteen years old, Tracy's had diabetes for a year. "It sucks, as far as I'm concerned. I'm sick of the rules, the restrictions, I'm sick of the scheduling, I'm sick of the shots, and—most of all—I'm sick of those yucky therapists. With all their agendas. And all this questioning about how I'm feeling, what I'm thinking about. Sure I'm ready to do myself in some days, so sue me why don't you?"

Sid steps into the center of the room, takes charge. "Okay, on your feet, time to act like you're having a good time. You don't have to tell me just how much of a good time you're not having. I get the message. Loud and clear. Let's see what we can do . . ."

He's caught them looking despite themselves. "Pretty weird dude," is the unspoken comment on the situation, "but maybe weird's better than the other thing." Sid gets them off their duffs and into a loose spaced-out circle around him. "Now, if you guys want to be performers—I mean if you want to strut the boards, you've gotta learn to breathe from your bellies—your diaphragms. Right here on top of your guts." He gets a few snickers from the boys; gut jokes always get them going. "Else you'll never be able to make the kind of noise you want to. Okay, I want to hear you project your voices so you can be heard on the tenth floor. No, I don't mean shouting, just let it come up out of your centers . . . out of your bellies . . . Right, you're getting it. . . .

"Okay, now we're going to play. Parts I mean. We're going to act—like we're having fun. Fake it till you make it, boys and girls, ladies and gentlemen. Okay, each of us is going to give their name and make a gesture that describes us . . . I don't care if it's obscene as long as it's the real you. . . ."

So they launch into the exercise, without time to ask themselves what the *expletive deleted* is going on around here. They're stubborn at first, trying to cover their embarrassment, their vulnerability, with more sneers and snickers. But pretty soon the peer pressure kicks in, and they're trying to outdo each other with outrageous actions and gesticulations.

Sid's after their *self-consciousness*—the actor's awareness of themselves as though they're seeing their reflection in a mirror. This is self-awareness of a productive kind. It's getting them to really see themselves right here and now, perhaps for the first time. It's getting them to start taking some real pride in their appearance *and* their performance.

Tracy's attention is caught up in the action. She thinks, "Hey, this guy's kind of cool. At least he's not asking me any f---ing questions. All he seems to want us to do is bounce around and make a bunch of noise . . . breathe with our bellies . . . cool . . . Hey, maybe he's a rock star from yesteryear . . . I'll breathe through my butt if he wants me to. . . ."

And so on. Sid takes these reluctant teenagers through several warm-up exercises that professional actors use to limber up their bodies and voices before a performance. Released from their real-life selves, they gradually begin to express themselves with a gusto they probably haven't felt since they were little tots. Until a few minutes ago a picture of self-pity and insolence, these young people are now transformed into colorful hams strutting their stuff for all to see. An astounding animation comes over everyone. It's both exciting and deeply moving. My heart goes out to them.

The Therapy of Drama

Sid isn't a professionally trained drama therapist. He's simply another artist, in this case an actor and director, who has taken his skills a step further and put them to work in the service of people with illness and disability. In prisons and hospitals, with some of the toughest audiences you can imagine, he's rarely failed to get his audience to participate. His approach seems to appeal directly to the urge deep within all of us to open up our imaginations through our bodies and their performance (Homan 1994).

He works with physicians and medical students too, giving them the actor's awareness of their bodily expression, especially in their interactions with patients. "If you have to go into a room and give someone bad news, what do you do with your body? Do you open the door confidently, or tentatively? Do you go and sit down before opening your mouth? How close do you sit to the person?" And so on: all nonverbal communication cues that are the stuff of theatre, and of real life.

The field of drama therapy was only recognized in this country twenty years ago, although it's been established longer in Europe. Social psychologist Erving Goffman (1961, p. 18) said this about its use in mental hospitals and prisons: "Since the staged circumstances of the portrayed characters are not the inmate's real ones, he has no need to exhibit distance from them." Drama therapist Renee Emunah, in her book *Acting for Real* (1994, p. xiii), puts it this way: "In the world of make-believe . . . we have the freedom and the permission to do what seems . . . so difficult . . . in life—to alter . . . role patterns. . . . Drama liberates us from confinement. . . ."

Perhaps the most creative and practical application of theatricals to everyone's education and health is the work of Keith Johnstone over the past forty years, first in London and gradually through his teaching about *improvisation* all over the world. In his book *Impro* (1992), he tells of how as a young man he unlocked his own spontaneous childhood creativity once more, and how he has since helped thousands of others to do the same. In her book *Writing Down the Bones* (1986), Natalie Goldberg, speaking of this natural genius within us, refers to the old Buddist concept of *beginner's mind*. Keith Johnstone teaches that art of all kinds is already in us; it doesn't need to be evaluated, imposed on, or meddled with. Developmentally delayed children are often the best pupils for this, he says, because they never get to take in all this adult conditioning that affects most of us from so early in life.

Exercise: Object Naming

Here's a simple exercise adapted from Johnstone's book. It's great to do with a partner, or best of all with several. First I must warn you though: It'll probably seem pretty silly to you at first, but all the best acting exercises are silly.

Okay. Put down this book and put aside whatever you planned to do next. Bring your mind into the room, or into the space you're in, fully, please. Open your eyes wide and look around. If you can, start pacing about. Look for just one instant of time at everything that comes into your line of vision.

Now start shouting out the *wrong* name for every object your eyes light upon. You're looking at familiar, and therefore normally unnoticed, everyday objects—chairs, windows, carpet, bed, ceiling, radio, washbasin, doorknob, and so on. So give them all everyday, but wrong, names. Call everything by the name of a vegetable, or an article of clothing, or something you'd see in the street.

You'll quickly find that this is not only silly-seeming, it's hard to do. It may help you if you point at each item your eyes light on as you name it. Try to keep mixing it up, staying spontaneous. Empty your mind. Don't rehearse. Be as quick as you can. Try not to think or even pause. Hurl a new name at each object. You'll splutter a bit, your mind will *lock up*, you'll even chide yourself that you can't think of a single name for something other than its *proper* name. Just keep spitting out those nonsense names, as fast as you can, as you stare intensely but momentarily at each object in turn. Keep as straight a face as you can, as an actor has to do when on stage. But if you and your partners have to burst out laughing, that's just fine too.

Twenty objects will do it. Okay, so how was it? Hard? Funny? Crazy? Easier as you got into it? Now look at everything in your range of vision again. Take a good look around. How do they appear, these familiar objects? More colorful? More sharply defined? A different size from before? More *interesting?*

Lifting the Veil of Unawareness

Anyone who does this exercise with gusto will have a transforming experience. Even the size and shape of the room may seem to have changed, because all at once you've brought commonplace things into full focus. You've lifted the veil of unawareness and inattention that, in our everyday encounters, separates us from the world around us. And this is a world that includes everyone else.

The truth is, we're seldom fully present and *here* for each other. We're rarely present in the way that babies see the world all the time—in a full-frontal, unveiled way, so much so that they have to learn to screen things out to to avoid sensory overload. The sad thing is that as a society we've taught our young to go to the opposite extreme. We've taught that dull, colorless, drab, boring is the nature of our minute-to-minute, day-to-day surroundings. So as our young ones grow, they increasingly start to *check out.* They disappear into themselves and their fantasy worlds where we can't follow.

Fantasy is not only wonderful, it's essential. But we need to be prepared to share it, and our real selves, with each other. We all need to stop drawing such a distinction between fantasy and reality. Because in sacred truth, the reality is *fantastic.* Take a look around. Things still look sharper, more colorful, don't they? Take a good long look at everything your creator has given you. And start to count your many blessings once more.

Exercise: Magic Ball

So here's another simple-silly exercise to do with a partner. You'll be exercising your acting skills to create totally imaginary objects to give to each other. (I've adapted this from the work of drama teacher Bernie Warren, 1997.)

One of you starts with an imaginary magic piece of modeling clay, which you start to roll around in your hands, shaping it into a gift for your partner. You can pull it any direction you like, molding it to fit your every whim. Because it's magic, you can let it expand in your hands as you shape it into a special present for your friend. Once you're entirely happy with what you've created, pass it across to them—taking care that it doesn't fall and perhaps shatter—with the appropriate gesture of giving.

Your partner will of course receive it with delight and appreciation. Once they've admired it appropriately and sufficiently, it will be their turn to mold the clay back into a round ball and shape their own object as a gift to you in return. An extra element is of course that you have to guess the nature of the gift before you "unwrap" it. "Ah! It's a new nightie (or vase of flowers or box of chocolates or set of kitchen knives, or whatever): how lovely!" Don't forget to tidy up the wrapping paper.

And so on: You can perhaps give each other several gifts of quite different kinds. Most people include a pet animal that perhaps gets nervous and escapes, running around and hiding under the wrapping paper. This is of course a great game for children, but you'll find it excellent for getting your miming skills going, and for letting your imagination run. It's especially good for helping you let go of any conscious control, so your emotions take over—because this is a work of emotion as well as art you're creating each time. Let it express something of yourself that you want to show to your friend, but that may be hard to put into words. Of course neither of you will bring any criticism or judgment to this simple game.

The Art of Drama and Dance: What Have We Learned?

The modern field of drama therapy is pretty new. The National Association of Drama Therapy was only founded in 1979. Actually though, this is an ancient art, at least as old as the classical Greek temples of healing, and it probably has echoes of the ancient shamanic practices of prehistory. Some of the earliest modern work with drama and healing was that of Erik Erikson (1950), who showed how children spontaneously use dramatic play to express their internal emotions, especially conflicts, to achieve a sense of control and mastery over their situation, to try on new roles in new situations, and to problem-solve. This work went on to be refined by child therapists and educators as the basis of drama therapy. Gradually these techniques have come to be used to help adults with all kinds of illnesses and disabilities.

It's become clear that dramatic play is crucial to the process of thinking, learning, and healing. Acting is an extension of the healing art of storytelling, which I talked about earlier in this book. Your life, like everyone else's, isn't made up of just one story but lots of interweaving ones. Even though everyone has an essential self—let's call it your *essence*—you show different personalities or *play different roles* with different people.

Perhaps the best thing about play-acting, or drama therapy, is how it stresses wellness rather than illness. Many psychologists have caught on to this and advocated it for years. It asks of you that you stretch yourself to your full potential, showing all your diverse faces and facets. This is creative self-expression at its best. If you're someone who suffers from a chronic illness, it can be life-transforming to realize you can still live a richly healthy life despite physical restrictions. The use of drama lets you explore all kinds of human interactions in a safe and nurturing environment.

Exercise: Playing Doctor and Patient

Let's try another one with a partner. Choose just one partner this time, someone you can have fun with. Again, this will feel pretty silly at first, but it's vital stuff for perking up your self-esteem. It will sharpen and enrich your relationships with other people too. You'll learn about both verbal and nonverbal communication—sorted out and simplified, so you can hold a mirror up to yourself and to each other. These are essential life skills that perhaps no one thought it important to teach you.

Sit in two chairs facing each other. If one of you's in bed, that's fine too. But get as *straight on* to each other as you can. Now, you're going to exchange short sentences, alternating with one sentence each, back and forth. One will play the role of what is conventionally considered an authority figure, in this case a doctor. The other is going to play the part of someone usually thought of as a lower-status figure—a patient, let's say. This is a question-and-answer session, just as if you'd gone to consult your doctor about a problem.

The "doctor" is going to take a medical history, so she starts it off by asking the "patient" a relevant question, to which he will reply. The tricky and silly bit is that the doctor's first question must start with an "A," and the patient's first answer with a "B." The doctor's second question must start with a "C," and the patient's second reply with a "D." You just keep going down the alphabet.

It might go like this: "Are you hurting anywhere?" "Behind my left knee, doctor." "Can you show me exactly where?" "Doubt it—I can't reach down that far." And so on. Some of the letters at the end are hard, of course, so you can cheat a little with "X" by substituting "Ex" as in "Excuse me" or "Exceptional"—although "X-ray time, do you think?" works pretty well.

This is a funny game with a serious purpose: that of getting you to have a conversation with your friend that makes you more aware of how we all view *status* in our society. Everything we do and say, every intonation and inflection, in our day-to-day relationships is unconsciously governed from a very early age by status. We're either *higher than* or *lower than*. To see this, try running the exercise again, but this time put into your expression as patient a deferential look— avoiding eye contact, looking down, perhaps shrinking into yourself. Now, as doctor, puff yourself up a bit and speak with assertion, even impatience, as though you're in a hurry. (I hope you've never had that experience with any doctors you've known.)

Okay, now you're going to *reverse* this process. Let the doctor become the nonassertive shrinking violet (I know, it's a bit of a stretch) and the patient the dominant, even demanding, one, expecting her demands to be met instantly. Try it with your nonverbal behavior first. Once you've gotten that down and have stopped laughing—you don't have to go right through the alphabet again— try changing the sentences a little bit. Add an "er" or an "um" to each of the doctor's questions, for example, to add even more diffidence and deference. Certainly changes things, doesn't it?

Now, even more interesting, one of you try drawling out those "er's" and "um's" some, and notice how it transforms them from being expressions of hesitancy to ones of controlling the dialogue once more. Instead of sounding like a mouse with a short timid "er," you start to sound like a wise owl with your deeply considered "umm-mmm," reminiscent of Wol the owl in the Winnie-the-Pooh books. By the way, the owl didn't know what he was talking about—quite a lot of people use such drawling as a cover-up for uncertainty. Perhaps you'll be back to sounding more like the real-life doctor once more.

There are endless variations on this exercise, so play around with it. Come back to it. Change the setting and the situation to a checkout line, or to asking directions of a stranger, or to being teacher and pupil in a schoolroom. Try different intonations: ones of deep curiosity, of boredom, of hilarity, and of romantic love. Make it as incongruous as you can, like making a romantic come-on out of paying off your taxi driver outside an airport. You might try hamming it up into a clown act when you ask your spouse a series of questions about what she'd like for dinner tonight. Play with both the verbal and the nonverbal.

"The Play's the Thing"

Because—to play on Shakespeare's famous words a little—if it's true that all the world's a stage, and all the men and women merely players, then all of life can be thought of as a play. Or you might say simply *play*. It's no accident that the word "play" has two different but allied meanings. A play is performed or acted out in a mostly pre-planned and heavily rehearsed fashion. Play (minus the indefinite article), on the other hand, is a spontaneous and improvised activity that you indulge in instinctively from earliest childhood. Unlike a play, it has no set beginning nor end, no curtain up nor final bow. And in your life you get to have your entrances and your exits, sometimes coming back onto stage many times. But always—even after your last line is spoken in the play and you've left the stage—you get to return for a final bow, and be the center of attention at your funeral or memorial service.

You see how closely you can apply this analogy to a person who is ill or in the hospital. When you're ill you're essentially alone, with your symptoms and the thoughts and feelings they bring up, which no one else can fully experience. Yet you're also center-stage as the patient, getting the kind of attention you might not have had in years. Would it surprise you to learn that, much as none of us deep down inside wants to be ill, or to die, some people quite enjoy the extra regard an illness brings? It's understandable though if you stop to think about it. When a little boy scrapes his knee falling off his new bike on the driveway, and asks his mom to kiss it better— or if he's too big for kisses, to hear him out as he bravely tries to stifle his tears—he experiences physical pain simultaneously with the delightful balm of emotional comfort blended into the mix. The contrasting mix of feelings this brings is just one of life's awesome paradoxes.

Of course, not all the consideration you get when you're ill is welcome. Many tests and treatments, including surgery (performed in the operating *theater* by the way), are painful, both physically and emotionally. Sometimes it seems in this modern age that doctors must first do harm in order to give help. Look at the many unwanted or so-called *side effects* of chemotherapy drugs given to patients with cancer as one example.

In the English theater, the topmost and so furthest away rows of seats were traditionally called "The Gods." Actors are always urged to project their voices and performances out to these members of the audience who are sitting furthest away in the back of the theater. So how can you best occupy center stage and project your voice and presence? How can you offer—project—your best performance, whatever your circumstances? So that when you take your final bow it will be to rapturous applause?

Exercise: Play-Acting—A Metaphor for Living

Now you're going to make a little play of your present life circumstances. Even if you're not suffering from an illness or similar problem, this will be an excellent way to see how you can take charge of your circumstances if you feel the need to do so. The patient, or the person in need (all of us at some point, make no mistake about it) depends a lot on others, just as the actor does. They call this group effort an *ensemble* in the theater. And ministering to the sick person is an art, whether you're a doctor or a nurse or a social worker, a psychologist or a chaplain or a cleaning lady. So equally is being sick or disabled an art: that of accepting it and performing your part to the best of your ability. Life is just one long piece of performance art.

So imagine you're going to be on stage tonight, as the lead actor or actress, and it's *opening night.* You're going to pick a piece out of your life, preferably your recent or current life, to enact as a play. And you're going to play to those gods watching from afar—from the back of your particular theater—as you perform your part in this play of life. This is what it's all about, to do your best by your creator—your director. If it helps make you a little less nervous on opening night, remember life is just a test, not the real thing. Otherwise they'd have sent you better instructions.

Take out your workbook and jot down ideas about this personal play of yours. You've been getting some practice in made-up conversation, so now let's turn it into a short three-act play with a beginning, a middle, and an end. It can be very short, with less than a page of lines for each act. You can make it a comedy or a tragedy, a soap opera or a thriller, but give it a happy ending. Start with a small cast of characters: say, yourself as the patient, with at least one of your closest family members or friends, and at least one caregiver (perhaps a doctor or nurse) as additional characters. If someone close to you is ill, then you can build the play around them. It's good to make this as true to your real-life circumstances as possible. Think about when you or your loved one got ill, or imagine such a scenario. This will be the *first act.* Write a few lines of back-and-forth conversation with the family members or friends, and perhaps bring in your first visit to the doctor. About a dozen lines or so of dialogue will do fine.

Then make the *second act* the central piece of the drama. Perhaps you have to come into the hospital for surgery, or many more tests. Write some lines of conversation with the doctor or nurse, and then with your family talking about all this drama, making those lines full of action and emotion. Keep everyone in suspense about the final outcome. Again, a page of dialogue will do fine, but keep going if it spills over onto another page or even two. Then come to the *final act,* the resolution of your story. Make sure you bring everyone in here, and—whatever your true-life circumstances that you're basing your play on—make this a happy outcome for everyone. Let the dialogue reflect this.

Now it's time to put your play on the stage. Remember, you're the playwright, director, *and* leading actor or actress. This is your play and your life, after all. First you need to cast the parts. Once again you'll need friends or family to help you, although if you have a friendly caregiver available who can give you some time, then that's ideal. It's best if you copy out the lines on two or three sheets, so you have several copies. You don't have to learn your lines; reading them out loud is just fine. If you want to gather a few props—a stethoscope, some bottles of medicine, a gown, a white coat, or even a bedpan—that just adds to the fun. You can use just one area for your play's performance, and you might want to add a little scenery—something that indicates that the first act takes place at your own home, for example. Make sure you signal the start and finish of each scene by a ritual, perhaps a little announcement to your audience.

Your audience can be just you performers—an audience of yourselves—but if you feel bold enough, you might want to perform your play again for a specially invited audience. When you come to read your lines, make sure you put plenty of feeling into them, and urge everyone to really get into their parts. Always speak up: remember, you've got to be heard by The Gods. If it feels right, you can ham it up a bit. You can change the cast of characters around too, perhaps having men play the female parts and vice versa. But remember that although hilarity is just fine, and will help you overcome the shyness you may feel as performers, this is a serious subject with serious intent. Seeing this piece of your life from the perspective of a play helps you step outside the real-life drama and even have a little more control over the way your life's unfolding. Keeping things a little lighthearted helps deal with any heavy theme, which this is likely to be, as it's dealing with illness that is close to home for you.

Tragedies and Comedies

This idea of turning life into a piece of performance art is at the core of how being an artist can help you with whatever affliction or calamity may affect you or your family members. The art of acting parts can become your friend, as faithful as any dog to its master. It really can serve you, just like Curt's journal served him in chapter 5. It's all about *reframing* things, to use a word that's popular with psychologists nowadays. This simply means looking at a situation differently. Sometimes I say to a dying person who has made it clear they're open to a little gentle humor: "Well, if you are going to die, I guess you'll just have to settle for life everlasting a bit earlier than me." That's a reframe, and one about which you can say, "There's many a true word spoken in jest."

You might call such reframing turning a tragedy into a comedy. It doesn't take away the tragic elements, especially for those left behind to grieve. But remember how close are tears and laughter. Haven't you ever heard laughter at a funeral wake? It's not at all uncommon for a recently bereaved person at the graveside of a beloved family member to feel a fit of the giggles coming on. The playwrights Shakespeare and Shaw were as proud of their comedies as they were of their tragedies, because they knew each had elements of the highest art. Many actors say it's harder to play comedy than tragic parts. The same applies to the painter Picasso—much of his work is humorous, interspersed with paintings of the deepest gravity. The tragic and the comic in art are simply two equally shining faces of the gemstone of human intelligence.

So reframing is another way of looking at things. If you can achieve such a perspective at a time of suffering—to see that all suffering is ultimately temporal—or temporary—you may well feel a sense of enormous relief. This is what the successful artist achieves. I hope by now you've felt the benefit of putting your story down on paper, or of acting something out, or of collaging it, or of whatever art form you've brought to bear on a given situation. This is why art can be life-saving. We can't survive as a human species without it, nor were we meant to.

Self-Consciousness Is Fine!

Performance art is mostly associated with a stage and an audience. But just as doodling and collage-making and journal writing can be for your eyes and ears only, so it is with performing. That's what an actor's or a dancer's or a stand-up comic's rehearsing is all about. Perhaps you can think of times when you went over, either in your mind or out loud, what you were going to say to someone when you had a potentially angry conversation ahead of you, or how you were going to behave after you got through telling a friend some bad news. But you'd probably have felt a bit silly, even embarrassed, to have been surprised in the act of doing just that—in the act of rehearsing, because it makes you self-conscious.

But self-consciousness is a vital part of living your life to the fullest. It's when you're *allowed to make mistakes*, so you can learn from them, and not make any—or not so many, anyway—when you do the actual performance. Imagine having to learn to play the violin from scratch in public. Children have no problem with this concept. They're happy to learn by falling on their well-padded bottoms for most of their first year out of the womb, to the adoring delight of their adults. And what stupendous applause they receive when they at last make it on to two feet. "Ah! Hurrah! Who's a clever girl then?"

Performing is something we all learn to do naturally. Mostly you do it without realizing it, unless it's drawn to your attention, often in a disparaging way. But there's good scientific evidence that such performing, whether it be through learning to dance or through playing the fool—dancing or clowning around spontaneously and outrageously—is good for your total health (Robinson 1991). For example, dancing can be enormously effective in relieving anxiety and stress. And the world's waking up to the therapeutic power of play. Behaving as children is sometimes good for us, even when chronologically we're aging adults.

On with the Dance

Are you one of those folks who think you can't dance? Most people are. Perhaps you even think that only *some* squirrels and kittens can dance, just like only *some* sparrows or nightingales can sing? The truth is: If you can speak you can sing, and if you can move you can dance. By dance, I don't necessarily mean moving your legs and feet to a definite, predetermined pattern of steps. Even if you're paralyzed from the waist down or both your legs are in plaster casts, you can still dance with your arms and wrists, your hands and fingers. Professional dancers would never dream of dancing only with their lower limbs. And even if you're paralyzed all the way from your neck down, then you can dance with every part of your face: your forehead, eyes, and eyebrows, your mouth and nose, your cheeks and chin, even your ears. And you'll be able to choreograph a pretty original dance too.

Choreographing is the name given to composing a dance piece or routine. It's just like composing a piece of music, or a score. In case you wondered, you actually compose subconsciously all the time, for example every morning when you move from bed to bathroom to toilet to closet to sock drawer to refrigerator to stove top (or microwave) to breakfast nook to kitchen sink (or dishwasher) to front door. You have a similar ritual of movement—of dance—even if you're waking up each day in a hospital bed. You're probably not thinking of it as a dance, though.

And every time you offer an expression of delight or surprise, fear or disgust, you compose a little routine that is deliberately expressive, through movement as well as voice, of your feelings at that moment. You see, dance is at its simplest level a statement of emotion. For people with disabilities, simple dances can be a marvelously liberating way to self-expression and self-healing. Dancing is good for your circulation, your balance, your fine muscle control, and not least your sense of self-esteem and mastery. But it's the emotional component contained within such art-making through movement that lifts it above exercise or physical therapy as a personal creative statement.

In all these actions, or *compositions*, you use a huge variety of muscles, voluntarily but automatically, if that isn't too much of a contradiction in terms for you. At some level you *choose* how to perform these actions. And you never do it the same way twice; it's a new composition every time. That's all dancing is at its simplest—moving muscles in rhythm, and with emotion—with *or without* musical accompaniment, aware or unaware. Do you think a child is aware of all the dances he does around the house, down the street, in the playground, back home again, every day? You've been there, remember?

Exercise: Moving to the Rhythm

So that's what you're going to do now: Compose a dance. Only you're going to bring to bear a little more consciousness than you usually give to it. You're going to focus your awareness on the use of all these beautiful muscles of yours. You don't have to write it down like some sort of elaborate musical score. You're going to make it easy as pie. You'll need your notebook, but only for recording all that happens, and how you felt about it.

Okay, let's limber up. This you're going to do mentally: It's left-brain stuff. If you want to do it in front of a mirror, that's ideal. But you may feel silly and uncomfortable about watching yourself, because you're going to awaken your self-consciousness once more, and you know what that can do to a person. So you don't have to watch yourself with your actual eyes, but watching yourself with the inner eye of your imagination is essential. That's what becoming aware is all about: seeing yourself within your body as it moves and has its being.

Take an actual and mental look at your whole self. If you're in bed, peek under the bedclothes as you mentally move down your body. Please see yourself with the eye of deep compassion, of self-forgiveness, for any imperfections that you may perceive. Remember, and affirm, that your body is beautiful, perfect, and intact in God's eyes. So see it with the eye of your creator. You are elegance personified: a mover, a shaker, a dancer, a poem-maker.

If you have access to music, especially music of your own choosing, pick out a cassette or CD you like. It can be any sort—it absolutely doesn't matter. Because any music, by definition, has rhythm. So pick a rhythm, a tempo, a beat, a volume, that you think you'd like to dance to. If it's early and you're still waking up, or you've just finished a big sleepy-making lunch, you might try a lively rhythm that will get you moving and shaking and energized. If it's late in your day and it's been a tiring or nerve-jangling one, then make it a slower, quieter rhythm that will settle you down, so you can sleep restfully.

Once you've got the music going, and have adjusted it to the volume that suits you, close your eyes and start to move. Start with your facial muscles, not quite at random but with some consistency and rhythm, keeping time with the music. Try raising your eyebrows half a dozen times, then wrinkling your nose from one side to the other. Now rhythmically close and open each eye in turn. Try pouting out your lips with similar frequency and rhythm. What are you smiling at? Are you asking yourself, "Is this dancing, is this art?" Be assured that it is. I told you you could do it.

And just think, you really are giving your face a workout, no kidding. If you don't believe me, keep this routine going for two or three minutes, then compose your face into complete stillness. Now notice that it feels different: a little warmer, a little tingly. Maybe it feels a little tired and achy, but certainly less stiff. This is exactly what physical workouts—aerobics—are all about. Think back to some earlier time in your life. Isn't this how you felt in your body as a whole the last time you really got down and tripped the light fantastic? It's just that you don't think of it as dancing if you're not moving your feet.

So now you're going to move the rest of your body. Move whatever parts you can, if you have some restrictions. Don't beat up on yourself if there are some parts where you notice a lot of stiffness and rustiness, feel creaking and groaning. This is all the more reason to oil that creak and bop that crunch: you'll soon be capering with the teenyboppers. If you manage to get up on your feet, fine—start swaying to whatever beat you've got going on the tape or radio. Now that you've gotten into it, you might want to up the tempo a bit. If your legs are out of commission, start working your arms, wrists, hands, fingers. There are countless patterns you can weave with them. You might want to watch, in the way you've watched dancers on the stage or the movie screen. See how sinuous and sultry you can be, like you're dancing with your beloved, and there's no one there to see. Or get jerky and syncopated, if you're listening to a rock or jazz rhythm. Just let your imagination fly.

The Primal Effects of Movement

Okay, you can unwind and relax: It's time to take stock. Are you feeling any different? Chances are you found yourself a little reluctant to stop, to put an end to the rhythm that you'd gotten into. You may just be feeling a little lift, a little jazzed, but in a nice way. If you were sleepy before you started, then you're probably less so now. You may well be feeling more alert and ready to tackle some more serious project or mental exercise. If you were just getting ready to settle down to sleep, and you kept the movement a little on the quieter side, it's likely you'll be all the more ready to close your eyes.

You benefit from moving in rhythm because it's a natural and much neglected activity that promotes the health of your body, mind, and spirit. It helps free you of fears and anxieties, boredom and sadness. It literally lifts your spirit in the way that religious chanting or singing can do. Most religious traditions, particularly in developing countries, use dance for such purposes. Jesus Christ was a great exponent, but we've neglected his teaching in this regard. For the !Kung bushmen of the Kalahari Desert, the weekly all-night dance is a personal, family, and community healing event, addressing the full range of bodily, emotional, and spiritual ills. This celebration is seen as integral to the tribe's other activities, not separate from them.

Dancing elevates and energizes your mental state. You find yourself thinking more clearly, ready to wrestle with an issue that was really bogging you down before. Ever heard of stretch breaks during long meetings? We just tend to be a little too inhibited to turn them into spontaneous dancing sessions and really make them count.

Exercise: Your Body's Messages

Here's another exercise, adapted from drama teacher Bernie Warren, that will help you become aware of messages from your body and give them expression through a simple dance. It will also help you appreciate the difference between movement as exercise and movement as dance, the latter being something that you use to communicate to others and to express yourself.

You can stand, sit, or lie down, depending on how able-bodied you are. Start by listening to your breath passing in and out of your lungs. Become aware of the different parts of your body, their level of comfort or discomfort, any physical aches or pains, and any emotional tensions. Find a central place of balance in your body and try to stay attentive to it. Now let yourself become aware of your body's weight on the ground, the bed, or the chair. Feel its heaviness and the strength of support beneath your buttocks and against your back.

Start to imagine a cushion of air in the spaces between each vertebra of your spine, as though it were buoying you up and allowing your back to expand. Start to move your body in small rotating movements around this central pivot, moving back and forth and around, making simple shapes in the air. After a few minutes, imagine a shape or gesture that fits with your body's energy, and form that shape in your movement. Let this be your own dance gesture. Repeat it until you have a memory of it—your personal dance signature. There you are: You're both a choreographer and a dancer.

Story: Jack Improvises

At fifty, Jack thought his active life as a golfer was coming to an end. He'd been getting out to the links very little recently, and now he couldn't imagine ever playing again. It seemed he was heading for life in a wheelchair.

A few months earlier, he'd started getting aches and pains in his lower back. They'd quickly spread to involve his shoulders and hips, feet and fingers. He'd felt a general lack of energy too, so he put it all down to a bout of the flu. But when things didn't pick up after a couple of weeks he sought help from his local doctor, who ran some blood tests and X-rays. He felt a little better after taking the ibuprofen his doctor prescribed for him, but it was very temporary. When he went back the following week, his doctor told him the tests suggested he had something going on that was more than a casual health problem. It looked like he might have rheumatoid arthritis or lupus.

These conditions are what is often called *autoimmune*, that is to say they arise from some unexplained flaw in your immune system, which for some mysterious reason starts making proteins called antibodies in the blood, directed against many of your own organs. This shows itself in several ways, and while the symptoms can mostly be relieved, it's at the expense of having to take drugs with their own side effects. These illnesses can't be cured, as far as we know.

Jack's doctor suggested an early appointment with a rheumatologist. The specialist suggested the best thing was for Jack to come into the hospital for a full assessment. After many more X-rays and what seemed like blood tests several times a day, the specialist confirmed the diagnosis of systemic lupus erythematosus (often shortened to SLE). Not only were many joints involved, but there were early signs of Jack's kidneys being involved. The doctor was very straightforward. "This is an incurable condition, and sometimes the kidneys can get very severely affected. They may even cease to work well enough to keep you alive. If that happens you'd need to be on dialysis, and even be a candidate for a kidney transplant. But the main thing right now is your joints. Actually, it's really your connective tissue that's the problem—the fibrous stuff that connects all of your body parts together. We can make a great deal of difference to your symptoms, but it'll mean taking several drugs, and they can have a lot of unwanted side effects."

All of which gave Jack a lot to think on. He decided that this doctor, even if he was pretty blunt, knew what he was talking about. But he wasn't ready to hand over all control to him. He'd been told he had an incurable illness. Okay, but surely there was a lot he could do for himself. He'd been letting his body go in recent years; maybe that's why he'd gotten sick. Working at the office long hours, stressed out by recent personnel changes, he'd let his golf go completely.

Right then and there he decided to take up ballroom dancing. Actually, this wasn't quite as spontaneous as it sounds. His wife had been after him to try it with her for a while, and had even researched the best teachers in town. "Hot damn, this is my perfect chance, just when everyone's telling me I'll have to put my poor old arthritic feet up and start a regimen of pills that if they don't make me impotent will certainly make what remaining hair I have fall out." A devilish little imp in Jack peeked out and said: "I'll show 'em . . ."

And so he did. He wasn't cured overnight of all his ills, even his arthritis. Nor did he stay rebellious about the medications the doctor prescribed. None of us will ever know if his attempts at dancing made any difference to how limber he was, or simply helped him forget his troubles for a bit and gave his marriage a shot in the arm at the same time—let alone whether it made any difference to the course of his lupus. But he's in a remission of his illness now, and still dancing, pretty clumsily it seems according to both him and his wife (I don't know what his instructor has to say).

But he says it's less frustrating, and less expensive, than golf. He's back at work and happy, he says, in a way he wouldn't have understood before he got ill.

Every Cloud Has a Silver Lining

For me, this is a great story about the *transformative* effects of illness. No one would wish this chronic and crippling illness on Jack, any more than cancer or a heart attack. But ask people with severe illnesses or disabilities, and it's a rare person who can't find something positive to say about the experience. Even if the body suffers, often the mind and spirit find compensation—balance—in the situation. No one knows why our creator made disease, and its accompanying suffering, alongside all the things of joy and beauty on this planet. But Jack and his wife certainly seemed to find some purpose in his situation. Although if the purpose of illness is to slow us down, it didn't seem to have that effect on him.

I was especially struck by Jack's resilience, his unwillingness to just give up and put himself metaphorically, or literally, to bed, under the weight of such a baffling and potentially crippling disease. No one could blame a person for being engulfed by helplessness and frustration, even self-pity, at such a turn of events. Yet it's often through physical affliction or injury that you seem to come to a realization of resources within yourself of which you were unaware. You might choose to give some extra attention to your body today, or this week, especially if you are one who rarely does so. Why not see yourself as a dancer, a performer, with your own share of rhythm and agility, style and grace?

8

Laughter and Play

The most revolutionary act is to decide to be publicly happy.

—Patch Adams

Inner Children: The Art of Play

In this chapter we're going to take a look at the art of play and laughter for healing's sake. There's a wonderfully expressive word, *galumphing*, that is very apt here. It means having harmless and aimless fun, just for its own sake. This is an art form that has been much neglected until recently, at least among adults. I'll review with you some of the research on the value of playing and having fun as a health-promoting activity, just like you used to do when you were very young. Keep in mind that there's a crucial distinction between humor that is unifying and nurturing and that which is hurtful and distancing. Unfortunately, we've learned as grown-ups to *turn off* our full and free expression of the happy side of our natures. Yet it's vital we reclaim this natural facility, especially at times of serious illness.

You can use laughter and play to help deal with physical illness and suffering, as well as the strong emotions like fear, anger, embarrassment, and grief that these adversities often evoke.

Story: Joey

Joey was eight when I last saw him, a Tennessee soldier boy with all his faculties honed. We were sitting together in my windowless eight-by-ten office on our hospital's bone marrow unit. I can still picture him: perched on the edge of the couch, thigh-to-thigh with his mom, his dad on an upright chair leaning back against the door, with me and Nancy, my nursing colleague of many years, facing them at close distance.

We were there to talk about his death, which seemed imminent. When his mother learned Joey's cancer had advanced out of control, that my best counsel was for them to take him home to Knoxville to the care of their family doc, she'd said to me at once, "I want him to know everything up front. I'm not going to hide anything from him. But can you tell him? I don't think we can do it."

So Joe was sensing the tension in the room, knew something was up. His eyes saucerlike, he was going to catch every word. I beat around the bush for a bit, then finally got to it: "Joey, you're going to die, go to heaven." My words were at once lost in his howl, just like a wolf's, and the hurling of his frail little body into the recesses of his mother's dress.

This went on for several minutes. We were all hushed, eyeing each other in panic. Then the silent tears came, from each of us. "Whatever else was right to do, this wasn't it," was the unspoken thought. Then just as suddenly, on a long-drawn-in breath's end, he stopped, swiveled out from the sanctuary of his mom's dress, spied the tears on each of our cheeks, and promptly decided that he'd done enough grieving for the moment. With the artistic and comic genius of eight summers, he knew just the thing to lighten things up around here. His eyes lit on the scattered paper mound covering most of the carpet around us—charts, photocopies, memos, journals—and he became in an instant the stand-up comic. Beaming at me, he demanded: "Didn't your mom teach you to pick up after yourself?"

The Therapy of Humor

This is the best example of therapeutic humor I've ever encountered. Joey's anguished outpourings of a few minutes before had quickly brought us all to our emotional knees. For him, though, it had served the transcendent purpose of a wholly natural libation—it had gotten him through the first onslaught of grief and fear and perhaps anger. It had brought him to a place where he could function flexibly, creatively, once more. Seeing the grief and helplessness of all the adults surrounding him, in that instant he had lifted us all on his broad artist's shoulders, by offering an eight-year-old's joke. After a moment of stunned disbelief that he'd actually made a joke, we all convulsed in laughter. I expect you've laughed until you've cried a few times—but what about crying till you laughed?

If you believe that God has a sense of humor—which seems likely since s/he invented humor—and scatters merry angels in your path to cheer you up at times of stress, then Joey was surely one of those angels. The creator of *Peter Pan*, J. M. Barrie, once said that when the first baby laughed, fairies were born. The word *humor* is Latin for "water," or "fluidity," reminding us of our primal origins in the womb. Children are natural humorists, comics, jokers, galumphers. They know the creative vitality of laughing, just as well as they know the value of play. You don't have to teach them about it, any more than you do about sucking on mom's breast when they're hungry. They come equipped with the message from above. It's simply us grown-ups who've *forgotten* it.

✒ *Exercise: Laughing Yourself into a Good Mood*

It may seem paradoxical at first, but the *best* time to laugh is when you feel *least* like it—that is, when you're sad or angry, fearful or embarrassed. Embarrassment is hardly a joyful experience. In fact, most of us struggle mightily to hide it when it strikes us. Yet what do you all do when it does hit you—when you're engulfed in that awful shame of making a fool of yourself? Right, you laugh. You can't stop yourself. "Silly me!" are the words that come most spontaneously to your lips.

So here's the challenge. However you're feeling right now, however sore, or down in the dumps, or out of sorts with the world, I dare you to *laugh*. Set yourself to giggling, without any promptings from jokes, cartoons, funny faces, or rude noises. You might have to start with just a titter, or even silent laughter inside if there are people around that you don't want to disturb or alarm. But just get right into it—fake it till you make it. Starting with a titter, move on to a snicker, then gradually pull your face into a bigger, noisier giggle. Try laughing with your mouth closed, although this might make you cough. To get yourself going, you could try conjuring up in your mind a time when you were thoroughly embarrassed. Most people can do that all too easily, even though they'd love to forget the occasion forever.

These kinds of tricks may well get you started because of their very absurdity. Then try widening and deepening this heartfelt experience into a cackle, working yourself up to a full guffaw. Finally, *reach for the belly laugh*. Well—are you laughing yet? Keep faking it. Believe me, you'll feel better. I know, you're worried about someone coming upon you, immediately calling it an emergency, shouting "the patient's gone bonkers, call the psychiatrist, put her in a padded cell." So, you can make this much easier on yourself by making sure you've got some privacy. You can even use a pillow to "hee-haw" and "yuk-yuk" into, especially when you reach the louder and higher registers. Then you'll only have yourself to be embarrassed in front of, although even that can bring up lots of discomfort. Don't worry, the discomfort is fine. If you're like everyone else I know, you've been hanging onto a lot of embarrassment for far too long. It's high time to have a hearty laugh and be rid of it.

Laughter as Inner Jogging

The whole point is that you never need a *reason* to laugh. If you think that laughing spontaneously, with nothing obvious to laugh at, is silly, even crazy, just think about children again. They do it all the time, until finally urged by their embarrassed grown-ups not to. The demand—"What on earth are you giggling at?"—will shut down a six-year-old's spontaneous laughter in an instant.

If you did manage to get into a good laugh about nothing at all, take stock of how your body felt. Did it feel a little out of breath, a little flushed, a little warmer, a little more *energized*? I hope you noticed something of the sort within you. *Saturday Evening Post* editor Norman Cousins—who in the late sixties learned the therapeutic value of laughing to relieve his chronic back pain—called laughter "inner jogging." This is an apt description for what is after all a form of aerobic exercise. He described in detail in his book *Anatomy of an Illness* (1979) how he used laughter, which he got started deliberately by checking out of his hospital room into the local hotel and watching Charlie Chaplin and Marx Brothers movies, to use it to reduce his chronic back pain and consequent insomnia.

People who have studied the physical effects of laughter have reported many beneficial things that it does to your body. These include deepening your breathing, and so improving the flow of oxygen through your lungs; improving your circulation, and so getting your blood flowing to almost forgotten parts; and relaxing muscles throughout your body, after first putting them through a thoroughly good workout (Fry and Salameh 1993; Goldstein and McGhee 1983).

Lessons from Children

Committing to laugh together *without justification*, except simply to help your body and mind and soul be healthier, is to seize your birthright of taking joy from every moment. The children I care for know the cardinal rule that Cicero so aptly stated: "Seize the day, put no trust in the morrow!" After all, as the playwright George Bernard Shaw pointed out, "Life doesn't cease to be funny when someone dies." Facing, like Joey, their own likely deaths, children will shed their tears, shake off their fears, and return to the present instant. Give them a little loving attention and they'll astound you with their courage and creativity. So you too can learn from children, and allow the baptism of humor's holy water to moisten both your tears and your laughter, to loosen your voice in song and your muscles and joints in dance.

The whole business of spontaneous laughter is much easier, and more effective, when done in the company of others. You just need a mutual understanding—*the* understanding—that this is very good for your health, because it is. Ever since Norman Cousins caught the world's attention by deliberately using laughter for pain relief and better sleep, we've been learning about its profound physiological benefits. Laughter is indeed the best medicine, as the *Reader's Digest* has been telling us for decades.

What exactly have we discovered about healing through laughter? What does it do for you? First, of course, it gets you *moving*. A moment's observation tells you you're working a lot of voluntary and involuntary muscles in your face and chest and belly when you shake with laughter. As I indicated earlier, research studies have shown that you get a good aerobic workout. Haven't you sometimes felt quite worn out with laughing, but in a relaxing and satisfyingly unwinding kind of way? It's been scientifically shown that it's impossible to relax one's muscles deeply and be anxious at the same time.

High Spirits and Your Physiology

A good guffaw brings your pulse and blood pressure down—after a very short-lived rise from all the excitement—and increases your blood supply to your distant parts, causing your skin temperature to go up. This certainly can't be bad if you suffer from poor circulation, or if you're on blood pressure pills. A recent study from a cardiac care unit reported that watching a funny video for as little as thirty minutes every day was enough to lower blood pressure and reduce heart arrhythmias and pain. Laughing hard gets you breathing deeper, opening up the often underused parts of your lungs, improving the supply of oxygen to every part of you, as Stanford University psychiatrist William Fry (1977) showed more than twenty years ago. Did you know a lot of us are not getting the amount of oxygen we really need, just because we don't breathe deeply on a regular basis? Fry calculated that laughing one hundred times is equivalent to fifteen minutes on a stationary bike.

Then there's the enhancing effect of laughter on your immune system—the vital cells and antibodies you create to resist every infection you'll meet throughout your life. This same system also plays a major part in eliminating cancerous cells from your body before they can get a hold and establish a visible cancer within you. Psychologist Herbert Lefcourt (1990) showed us that listening to a humorous tape significantly raises the antibody immunoglobulin-A in your saliva; this is your first line of defense against both bacterial and viral infections. Researcher Lee Berk (1989) and his colleagues have widened the scope of these studies by showing that lots of your antibodies and your body's other lines of defense are perked up by laughing freely. "Laughter is hazardous to your illness," concludes Dr. Berk.

Laughter and Your Brain

Perhaps the key to all these effects is how laughter affects your brain's working day, especially the hormones I've told you about called endorphins. These are the several dozen brain-chemical messengers of mood and behavior, or "molecules of emotion," as their discoverer Candace Pert (1997) calls them: chemicals that create all those familiar good feelings in you, like exhilaration, joy, love, satisfaction. They also purge you of those negative emotions—anxiety, depression, and boredom—"the blahs," as you might call them. Dr. Pert and other researchers have shown us that this link between expressing your feelings and releasing your endorphins happens not just in the brain but perhaps everywhere in your body. They can even reduce or eliminate your awareness of physical pain, which is why Norman Cousins found a Marks Brothers movie helped him get to sleep at night.

Story: The Food Fight

I remember my notorious seventh birthday party. I must have had about ten (though it seemed like a hundred) of my best friends, all boys, from school and the neighborhood over. There was a barely suppressed excitement in the air from the moment we got started with the huge birthday tea. After satisfying the edges of hunger, and after the adults had, praise be, temporarily withdrawn from our presence, came several glorious minutes of food-fighting.

The jelly and cake and icing and *blancmange*—even, amazingly, the Neapolitan ice cream—quickly started to fly through the air in all directions. Oh my golly, such pure freedom, such lack of restraint. We must have been unloading our missiles for many minutes, an infinite time of joy, reaching a crescendo of wild giggling and guffawing, when some especially soggy and splashy confection scored a spectacular hit against the lampshade hanging over the middle of the kitchen table, around which we'd been stuffing ourselves a few minutes before.

The cheers brought several adults running, among them my mother. There was a gradual restoring of order, during which we all had to help in the general cleanup. What I remember, to the undying credit of those several parents, is that we got off with fairly prolonged scolding. We weren't all sent home or to bed in disgrace. The party was even allowed to continue, once we'd all come to our senses—only with well-ordered and well-supervised games.

Exercise: A Childhood Memory

So this exercise is designed to get you back in touch with your spontaneously playful young-child self. You need a friend to do it with, but no other props whatsoever. It's even better to do this in a group, splitting into pairs and then coming back together to share your experiences.

Get comfy and make sure you won't be disturbed for twenty minutes or so. You might need longer; it depends on the size of your group. You're going to take turns listening and being listened to—"split time," I call it. The speaker gets five minutes to recall aloud any funny memories from their childhood, *the sillier the better*. Cast back in your memory for occasions of happiness that brought you closer to your friends. But it's especially not your purpose to remember moments of teasing or being teased, put-down joke-telling, or any other kinds of humorous occasions at the expense of others.

This avoidance of put-downs and laughing at others should include *yourself too*. Just because you're Jewish doesn't mean that telling an anti-Semitic joke is any more acceptable or will have any healing benefits. That we do tend to tell jokes against ourselves, often deeply unkind and self-demeaning, is just an extension of the socializing we've almost all of us learned well in our society. It's still very much part of the oppressive use of smirking laughter against others—just internalized within you, that's all. It has absolutely no positive value as a healing art, so I discourage its use. Often, the further you go back in your childhood, the gentler and sillier the memory will be. When you were very young you were less likely to have been contaminated by this conditioning.

Decide which of you is to be the listener the first time around, and which the storyteller. The rules are simply that the listener listens without interruption, and minimal prompting, while the speaker recounts a funny memory from his early childhood. Most importantly, if similar memories are stimulated in you by what you hear, just put them aside until it's your turn. Your task is to be fully available as a *listening post*, someone who can be relied on to pay good attention, and not laugh at the silliest or even most embarrassing memories. This doesn't mean you have to sit there with a deadpan expression on your face. Encouraging noises and eager smiles are fine, just don't interrupt the flow.

The task when you are the teller is to take your mind back, as empty and receptive as you can, to early childhood—the earlier the better. Free-associate with some links to your life at that time: siblings, buddies, school, and after-school activities. Try to focus on one incident. It doesn't have to be the funniest thing that ever happened to you, just something that comes back as a moment of uninhibited joy and fun. Then offer it up to your partner, and to yourself.

Paint as full a picture as you can. What were the circumstances? Where were you? Who was there? How old were you? What was so funny about it, if you can remember? Flesh out the details as much as you can. Recall just how you felt, and get right into that feeling of childish delight. Relish it as if it were happening right now. It can help if you tell your story in the present tense. Let yourself get into a hearty laugh at the memory, just as I do when I think of that slick and sticky birthday food splattered on the kitchen lampshade. Delight in yourself and your friends fully once more.

After about five minutes, switch over and see what your partner has to recount. Enjoy the memory with her, but be careful not to laugh at or interrupt her. Notice that these memories may evoke some tears too, even anger. Laughter is a gateway to each one of your emotions, so keep the atmosphere safe and receptive. Finally, if there are several of you, settle down to telling your stories together, sharing these hilarious memories of the art of fun and play.

Patch—and Other Evolutionary Probes

Patch Adams was the subject of the recent Hollywood hit movie of the same name. The "clown-doctor" says that *deciding to be publicly happy* is the most revolutionary act you can aspire to: It's a pie in the face, he says, of our society's dreadful conditioning toward pessimism, cynicism, and negativity. But it is a decision, just like deciding to laugh for no reason except that it makes you feel better. Patch hasn't been out of some kind of clown costume ever since his internship twenty-five years ago, when he left behind the conservatism of our medical establishment and struck out on his own. Ever since that time, he's given his doctoring skills away for free, earning his living by being funny and helping others do the same. His joyful and glee-filled philosophy has caught the world's attention ever since Hollywood decided to celebrate it in their box-office blockbuster, with Robin Williams playing Patch.

Patch's revolt has been from the start an *absolute* one against the *business* of medical care: "If you wanted a revolution and you couldn't use weapons but you had love, what kind of revolution would you create?" he asks. Every November he makes a pilgrimage to Russia with about thirty other clowns. He tells those who have little or no experience, and are nervous about exhibiting themselves: "That's fine—if you're shy, come as a shy clown."

A recent research study found that adults laugh fifteen times a day, while children do so four hundred times. Maybe this explains the difference in mortality rates. The eccentric Salvador Dalí once said: "I don't take drugs. I am drugs." But it shouldn't take life-challenging illness for you to put humor to work. Isn't it time we all put a stop to this epidemic of casual pill-swallowing to make us feel better: Valium and Tagamet and Prozac and the like? They all tend to quash our natural human feelings rather than encourage them. A dose of laughter should be prescribed several times a day on a regular basis—as a staple, not a luxury. There's a terrible *solemnity* pervading the care of the sick. It's a mix of grief that people feel too shy to speak of, guilt that the sufferer is so dependent on others, and fear of the unknown future. It's terribly limiting for our society to be, as writer E. B. White put it, "suspicious of anything non-serious." Such restraint is sillier than the silliest thing we could ever think of that would give our artistic genius full rein. It's really fine for you to fall on your face a lot, as long as you have others to pick you up and dust you off. It's the way you'll break down the false barriers between you and everyone else.

The Friendly Universe

The reality is, you *can* cope. You can bat out of the park every curve ball life throws at you. It isn't anyone's fault that you or anyone else gets sick, it's just God's will. But you can cry and you can

laugh—a lot of each—and feel much much happier as a result. You'll
also be far better equipped to deal with life's vicissitudes. The reality
is that the universe is here to help you, to do you *good*. It isn't an
unfriendly, hostile world out there trying to get you—quite the
reverse. Sadly, the great majority of people have been raised in an
atmosphere of mistrust, expecting difficulties and troubles as if they
deserved them.

Look at the way young children behave toward each other, com-
pared with adults. Infants and pre-schoolers, before it's been trained
out of them, will instantly befriend any newcomer, young or old.
They see the world as full of joy and excitement and fun adventures,
to be savored in the company of others. Older children and adults
learn the disastrous lesson that you mustn't instantly try to befriend
everybody, that you'll be taken advantage of or harmed if you do. So
in elevators on the way to our offices, we stand stiff and silent
amongst a throng of our fellow human beings, all facing to the front.
Start talking to everyone and you're labeled eccentric—somehow *not
okay*.

Of all the art forms, humor helps you rise above the stifling
training you got when you were young that taught you to obey the
correct protocol in dress, speech, and behavior. It will help you get
comfy with breaking these rules. You'll start to feel fine stepping out
of line, seeing the funny side in the world around you, sampling the
fruits of being a child again. In order to assert this authentic self of
yours, though, you'll need to get and give a helping hand—often. It's
hard to break out of conformity and have a downright good time
without a lot of help, which is why I put such stress on togetherness
in making art in all its forms.

I'm going to offer you a series of quick exercises that are pick-
me-ups for any occasion. They're especially good when you're feeling
blue or the person you're with needs lightening up. You'll probably
find one of these games more appealing than another, but try them
all on for size. Here we go . . .

Exercise: Why Be Happy? Why Not?

This is an exercise in pinning down one thing that—right now—
you're enormously happy about and grateful for. It will be helpful to
keep this light; don't make it too solemn. Sometimes even this little
assignment can be a stretch, when the world seems all at once to be
loaded against you, too much to cope with, gone to hell in a hand-
basket. I often do this exercise with staff before morning ward
rounds, and you'd be amazed how many want to pass when it comes
to their turn. But believe me, there's *always something to be happy about*.

Do this exercise with a friend or partner. If you're in a hospital, perhaps you can pick just one of the staff who has a bit more slack in their schedule and some free attention to give you. Then you can urge each other on when it seems really hard to identify anything at all to cheer you up. But don't prompt each other. The inspiration must come out of *your own* thinking and memory and intuition, and your own creativity.

You can certainly do this exercise on your own. If you do, use your exercise book to make a list of all the things right now that you're totally delighted with about yourself and the rest of your world. Remember though: Keep it light, so you don't get hung up on the more serious aspects of life. This is an exercise in the art of light humor. Your examples can be ever so simple and silly; in fact, they're the best kind. Here are a few to get you started. What about the fact that you've still got *some* of your own teeth, or that you can still taste chocolate, still go to the bathroom and clean up afterwards without help, or remember your friend's name on only the third try? Aim for about ten easy examples, and bend the rules a bit too. If you don't have any of your own teeth, try declaring with delight how utterly grateful you are that you did have them all for the first forty-three years of your life.

Got the idea? So let's go: What's one thing you're enormously happy about? *Enormously.* Go ahead and create your list.

Exercise: Laughing With, Not At

Remember (if you took Latin) that the word *humor* means "water," or "lubrication"? Water is something that helps things flow easily. It wasn't meant to make things more distant and sticky between us. The world-renowned musician-humorist Victor Borge said that "A smile is the closest distance between two people." Yet we've learned too well the evil art of put-downs that put distance between us and the object of our mirth—this is definitely not healing humor.

This exercise will put you in mind of how to use healing humor to build bridges, not barriers, between people. Again, it's ideal to have another person to try this with, but it isn't essential. List-making in your notebook, for later sharing with another, or with yourself when you're in need of a boost, is just fine.

Start to brainstorm: List in your notebook, in two columns, examples of both laughing *with* and laughing *at*. See if you can make a clear distinction, guided by the vital rule of using humor only for building stronger ties between yourself and others, at all costs not pushing them away. So, for example, humor that is lightly supportive is healing, while even the slightest kind of sarcasm is decidedly not.

Humor that includes others is healing, while that which deliberately excludes others is not. Laughing at the expense of a defined group of others—like overweight or Catholic or gay or children or deaf or old or Irish or Arab or people of any color other than your own—is definitely laughing *at*. Making a little light of a disability within a group of disabled people who have the same difficulty as you buttoning up their clothes or remembering someone's name is laughing with. Just be certain never to put yourself or anyone else down.

Again, try for a list of ten good examples. You'll find that as you develop these self-healing humor habits and put them to work, you'll get attuned to better and better examples. This is the nature of all art forms, and our own native genius for it. Practice makes for greater skill and success. Use it or lose it, as they say.

The Power of Invention

For some years now I've collected toys. For my fifty-seventh birthday I received nothing but goofy ones. We celebrated at a quite posh restaurant, and of course I didn't know what was in the boxes that wife and mom-in-law insisted I take with me to open over the desserts. It loosened up the slightly stuffy atmosphere to unwrap a bunch of squeaky stuffed animals and wind-up creatures of all sorts. We soon had these clockwork penguins and Kermits zooming between tables and tripping up the waiters.

By goofy I mean toys—props—that are funny in lighthearted and harmless ways, that need no words. They speak for themselves. How about finger puppets, bouncing balls that make funny noises, whoopee cushions, clown noses, goofy glasses, grinning cardboard lips-on-sticks, wind-up false teeth, and any manner of funny hats? I have about fifty hats of all shapes and sizes, many homemade by children and other playmates. I also find that since I started collecting these toys, people give them to me as gifts without any soliciting—and I'm not even ill or in special need. I just received in the mail, from a company marketing a new line of products, a pair of socks that have designed on them all the bones of the foot and ankle: anatomically correct, you might say.

It's one thing to collect these toys and bring them with you when you're going to the hospital, or to work, or to an appointment you're not relishing. It's a further stretch to put them to regular use. The important thing is that this very good habit gets easier with practice. Be willing to feel foolish at first when you don the clown wig or pull on a couple of finger puppets. Just get into it, and know that everyone else in the world is dying to make such a fool of themselves, to be really childlike once more. They're just too shy or embarrassed or caught up in life's solemnities to let loose and try it.

I often do what I call "Laughter and Play" workshops, where I give away a lot of red noses and other props. The only rule is that those who claim the noses have to be wearing them when they leave the workshop. Of course, once you set an example of *making a fool of yourself*, you can quickly recruit others to do the same, and make it a regular part of your support group's ritual activities to display your latest play-trophies.

Exercise: *Articulation*

Now for a couple of wacky games that any two or more people can play. They'll remind you of the games children invent all the time, and that stand the test of time because of their enduring funniness.

See if you can think of some funny tongue-twisting pseudo-medical phrases that are deliberately hard to say. These will be ideal to use with your friends or family, your doctor or nurse, next time they come around. The two rules are that they must be hard to say quickly, and you and others have to repeat them several times. Try silly symptoms like, "Ooh my abominable abdominals," or absurd therapies like, "I need my lemon liniment, my garlic gargle."

Here are a few more to build sentences around, or to practice repeating to each other ten times quickly: magical medicinal, terminal tomotomy, private prosthesis, hemorrhoidal hormones/hormonal hemorrhoids, bronchial proctoscopy, nutritious dishes, cardiac hysteria, medical maternity, plastic malpractice, hospitable hospitals, sterile stethoscope, alimentary allergy . . . and so on.

These are great tongue-twisters for getting you going in the morning. Pin up a list of them in large capitals in your art-making studio or cubbyhole, or on a board at the bottom of your bed for others to practice when they come visiting. Carry them around in your handbag or wallet for a few moments' sharing of complaints and procedures.

Exercise: *Galumphing*

Anthropologist Stephen Nachmanovitch adopted this term in his book *Free Play* (1990) to describe doing everyday, routine things in an unusual, harder, but funnier way. The word is one Lewis Carroll, the creator of *Alice in Wonderland*, made up.

You see this game being played not just by human children but by chimps and many other young primates. What you have to do is elaborate on commonplace actions to make them more interesting and playful. Children are forever inventing new ways to do *anything*.

A central property of art—whether it's music or poetry or painting or humor—is that it never takes the most direct route between two points. It explores the highways and byways of truth, seeking out and elaborating on its mysteries and nuances, alternates and charms. This is what many games are founded on. Why not take a longer or more devious route for a change, or try a more challenging, prettier way of doing things?

Apply this to any of the common actions of your daily life: getting dressed or undressed, going to work, or even dealing with the many aspects of an illness and its limitations. Try hopping rather than walking. Use your other hand or foot first. Change the order of doing a routine task like brushing your teeth or hair. Try doing things blindfolded, "trust-walking" while another person guides you.

Not only will this wake you up to greater awareness of the present instant, it will also make everything a lot more fun. We used to have an uproarious time when I was young (often accompanied by grown-ups, I'm pleased to say), running egg-and-spoon races. You had to race for the finish line while balancing an uncooked egg on a teaspoon. We also loved to run three-legged races. Several pairs of people competed in a footrace, each with one of their legs tied to another person's. Try doing that with a straight face.

This exercise is also best done in pairs or groups, but that's not essential. Getting yourself laughing and lightening up is the most vital thing, especially if you're having a hard time doing those routine things you never had to think about most of your life. You might try galumphing when, for example, you're getting dressed, or doing bathroom tasks, doing your hair or eating breakfast—especially if you already need help with any of these routine tasks. Just the simple switch of doing things with your non-dominant hand, or with your eyes closed, will do the trick of getting you present in the moment and giggling at how clumsy you are. If you're right-handed, try brushing your hair or buttoning your shirt with your left hand, and vice versa. Simply getting in or out of your bed from the bottom end will certainly cut it. See how inventive and funny you can be.

Exercise: Tantrums

Here's one more I've been using in group work for some years. I said earlier that you can use laughter to help lift you out of any fit of the blahs. This includes anger, which many people store up inside themselves as much as they do embarrassment. Once more, children set an excellent example. They know how to blow off their anger very fast and explosively, in the form of tantrums. If a three-year-old is allowed to express her feelings in this way instead of being at once scolded or otherwise restrained from venting her fury, she'll very quickly get over it and put it behind her. But we learn very early that it's *not all right* to express angry feelings, particularly for girls and women, so we're very unpracticed at it.

So here's your chance: Welcome to the tantrum mat. You're going to need a sheet of 8½-by-11-inch paper, or perhaps you'd better have several for future angry outbursts. You'll also need a bright red marker (red is a good color for anger). Place the paper on the floor and stand on it. You're going to trace the outline of your feet or your shoes on the paper. If you can't reach down to do it, either get someone else to help or just take a look at where the edges are and have a good try at tracing the outline. It's not crucial to be accurate.

That's it. Make a few spares while you're at it.

All you have to do is stand in the middle and jump up and down as fast as you can, shaking your fists and making as much noise in the form of incoherent screaming as you want to. Keep it up for at least a minute if you can, then take a breath, and go at it again if you're into it. You'll soon discover that, just like hearty laughter, having a deliberate tantrum is an excellent form of aerobic exercise. You'll get pretty breathless pretty quickly after a good tantrum or two. But I can assure you that you'll have those lovely endorphins jumping in no time.

Now, as with the expression of any other strong emotion, it's important to pick a suitable time and place. You may want to have someone to play this game with. They can trace their own feet and stand opposite you and do the same thing, as a dual act. But doing it alone is fine, in which case you'll want a bit of privacy. If it's hard to find a soundproof place, grab a pillow to clutch and scream into as you do your rapid up-and-down jumping.

Yes, this seems funny, and expect to be convulsed in laughter pretty quickly, especially if you do it with a friend. But I assure you that, as with all the best healing humor, you'll be doing this with serious intent. I said earlier that often when you're angry you can, if you set your mind to it, quite rapidly get to a place where you see the funny side of things. This exercise is a shortcut. I'm sure you have plenty of things happen in your daily life that irritate, even infuriate you. Well, this is a good way for you to blow off steam and the sources of your irritation at the same time.

Your Right Brain and Your Left

Not only is laughter a great way to shake yourself free of negative emotion, it also helps you get your thinking clear when you're confused, baffled, flustered, or have input overload. All these feelings can evoke anger and fear and embarrassment, each of which will definitely shut down your best thinking. This can happen a lot when you're sick, especially in hospitals, where you have to answer lots of questions, absorb tons of information, and make decisions.

The emotional outpouring that comes with laughing heartily doesn't just awaken your right brain—it helps your left brain do its stuff on cue too. It's those excellent endorphins, relaxing and invigorating you all at once. They loosen up your biochemical flow of information, let you take yourself and life around you a little less solemnly, and help you function at your peak. It comes down to simply putting your creativity to work in everything you turn your mind and hand to. What could be healthier than that?

9

Good Health to Your Body, Mind, and Spirit

If life isn't a great adventure, it's nothing.

—Helen Keller

Coming Back to Holism

In this chapter I want to return with you to the idea of holism—of wholeness—that I talked about in earlier chapters. I mean by this going after the health of your body, mind, and spirit as a whole piece, and striving to be in the best overall health you can in relation to other people and the world around you. When it comes to thinking about what links art-making to health, the spiritual element is the most vital of all. It's central to reaching and maintaining the very best physical, mental, social, and emotional health you're capable of.

But understand that by spiritual health I'm not talking about how many times you go to your church or synagogue or mosque each week. It doesn't even have much to do with religious attitudes or behaviors. Think instead about that *spirit* that you bring to an encounter or activity of any kind. It's no accident we use this word in phrases like: that's the spirit, a spirited performance, putting a lot of spirit into it, entering into the spirit of the thing, and so on. Then there's the other word that we use pretty freely in our language: soul—as in getting to soul of the matter, in my innermost soul, or baring your soul. Then of course there's soul music!

The Life Force Within You

If I were to define both of these words, spirit and soul, I'd say they refer to that central core of your being that gives you your energy and zest for life. In other words, it's your life force. Some people call this your innate healing power or energy. A word from traditional Chinese medicine that you'll run across sooner or later—because it's being recognized more and more as central to your total health as a human being—is *chi*. This is what the Chinese, actually Asian doctors generally, refer to as life force. They see it as flowing continuously throughout each one of us. It is this energy, which I like to think of as a great health-bearing breath of wind, that is thought to be interrupted when a person encounters illness or injury of any kind.

There are many medical and other approaches that have been developed in Asia over thousands of years to help free up this flow of chi within you when it's interfered with, so as to put you back into good health once more. These range from *tai chi* and *yoga*—ancient teachings that originally had a spiritual basis but are increasingly seen as beneficial to many aspects of your health—to acupuncture, which is at the core of many Asian medical systems. Acupuncture is also practiced widely in Western countries, as you may know, and has been shown in many scientific experiments to improve a wide variety of chronic medical conditions (Kaptchuk 1983).

Notice the emphasis that traditional Chinese medicine has always laid on health rather than illness. Chinese people used to only pay their physician when they were healthy, and would stop paying when they got ill, until the time they were restored to health once more. It's only in Western countries that we've gotten hung up with disease and what's *wrong* with you, rather than thinking about all the things that are *right* with you. This life force is tied inextricably to the creative instincts you were born with—the muse that remains alive and well within. Even if you've entirely neglected this innate art-making muse of yours since early childhood, you have nothing to worry about because it's still in there, dormant but intact, waiting to spring forth in the service of your health and happiness. It's waiting, if you will, to make music.

This infinitely creative life force isn't limited by any aging or physical wear and tear you may be experiencing. It has much more to do with your personal experience of inner harmony and contentment. It's also linked to your sense of control, even mastery, of the events of your external life. Making art is the fastest and best way I know of to reclaim your early childhood experience of awe and rapture, whatever may be your chronological age or bodily condition right now.

Exercise: Life Force

Try this exercise to see if you can identify, and locate, this life force within you. You can easily do this alone, indeed you may prefer to. But having a friend or a group to do it with is absolutely grand.

First, take a fresh page of your workbook and brainstorm as many words or phrases as you can that seem to describe it. I'll give you a few to get you started: vitality, lifeblood, animation, heart, liveliness, breath of life, inner reality, true being, divine spark, essence, inner core, driving force. Got the idea? Notice how many there are that describe essentially the same indefinable thing within you. Now see how many you can add to this list.

Okay? Now the *next* part of this exercise is to write a paragraph—no more, just eight to ten lines—that fleshes out these descriptive words and phrases as they apply to you. Start by breathing deeply in and out from your diaphragm a few times, to get yourself centered and focused. Now read through your list again. Notice what thoughts and feelings and images come to you. What part of your body are they coming from? Are they arising from your skin's surface—the junction between your inner and outer world? Or are they emerging from somewhere so deep that you're only barely aware of it? Start writing about this ineffable thing within you. It's within all of us, and in some way it unites us all together. Try not to think too much, just write as a kind of stream of consciousness. Go for your sense of awe and wonder at the very real power, the vitality, that is at the heart and soul of you, no matter what your outward bodily condition may be.

The *final* part of this exercise is to use other art forms to capture this same life force. Taking off from where you are now with your list-making and your writing, try to incorporate picture-making, sound, and movement. Take up your crayons or chalks and start sketching on a new page what this force you've conjured up looks like. You might want to draw a big outline of yourself first, then envision your chi flowing within you. What part of you does it occupy? How big is it? What color and shape? Get really bold with your lines, colors, shapes, and patterns.

Next, transform this drawing and writing into sound and movement. You may well find it easiest to close your eyes for this. Create a little dance of celebration of all your blessed and essential energy. Let your body move from wherever that core is located. You don't have to get up from where you're sitting or lying to do this. And above all, it doesn't have to make sense, even to you. Just let the rhythm of your whole being take you away. Then when you're ready, start to accompany this dance you're composing with a little song or a series of vowel sounds. Remember the kind of hums and thrums and chants and happy murmurings that I taught you about in chapter 6? Don't forget, *if you can talk you can sing. And if you can move you can dance.* Make it as quiet or as loud as you like, going up and down your vocal range as your spirit moves you. And make your movements as subtle or as boisterous as feels right for you.

When you feel you're finished, let your song and dance come to a graceful end. Take a bow or curtsy to your audience, real or imaginary, and accept the applause. Know that you have created for yourself, using several art forms all spinning off each other, the true *authentic* you. Don't forget to note the date and place, and anything that will trigger your memory later about your present thoughts and feelings. You can return to this life-force-bestowing exercise as often as you like. I encourage you to do so, because in "creating" this picture, this story, this dance, this song of yourself, you've expanded your self-awareness, and gone a long way to releasing any clogs and blockages you may have to the free, health-giving flow of your chi.

Story: Living a Full Life

Maurice was in his late sixties when I knew him. He'd just learned that he had widespread prostate cancer. His doctors had told him, very caringly but very clearly, that there wasn't much they could offer in the way of medical treatment. Because the cancer had spread to the bones of his spine and hips, he needed to take regular and increasingly powerful doses of medicine for the pain. He was also getting a series of hormone shots that offered some possibility of slowing down the course of the illness. That was it as far as medical science went. So aside from collecting refills on his prescriptions, he decided then and there that he had no more need of the medical profession.

Yet from the start Maurice seemed to greet the news of his illness and its probable outcome almost like a *license to live.* At the time of his diagnosis he was still working full-time as the head of a busy engineering business. He was pretty much a workaholic, so he hadn't taken a proper vacation in ten years. Like many busy people, he'd neglected his family in favor of long hours at the office. With the minimum of delay needed to hand everything over lock, stock, and barrel to his longtime business partner, Maurice announced his retirement and moved himself out of his office.

The first thing he told everyone—all his family members and friends—was that he wanted no long faces around. He was especially clear about any expressions of condolence or sympathy: He didn't need them. "If you can't be cheerful around me, don't bother visiting," he told people with his typical directness. Then he announced that there were a lot of things he wanted to do that he'd put off for far too long, and that he wasn't waiting any longer.

The first thing he did was to take up horseback riding. This was something he'd always yearned to do and, by golly, he wasn't going to let a few aches and pains get in his way. From then on, he rode two or three times a week, often full of strong pain medication, up until a few days before his death. He even learned to canter, and took a couple of falls that could easily have fractured several of his already weakened bones. And far from getting under his wife Dorothy's feet at home, he started to commandeer the kitchen, buying two or three gourmet cookbooks and teaching himself—with quite a bit of help from her—the utterly rewarding art of cooking. He tried out these increasingly delicious culinary experiments on a succession of friends and family, as well as himself, even catering several dinner parties.

He requested a visit from his grown son and daughter-in-law, whom he'd hardly seen in recent years, and urged them to leave his grandson and granddaughter with him and Dorothy, so they could get to know them better. This served as an excuse to go to Disney World and the other Florida tourist attractions they hadn't visited in years. Maurice remained mentally and spiritually vigorous—*spirited*—until the very end of his life. Almost exactly a year from the day that he'd learned he had cancer, his wife told me that it had been the best year of their thirty-year marriage, even though, or perhaps because, they were living under the shadow of it being cut short all too soon. Not only had they enjoyed all kinds of fun activities together with their family and friends, but they'd been able to find the courage and honesty to talk over the most important things in life today and in the future.

Exercise: Carpe Diem

Maurice's last year on Earth seems to me to have been a marvelous example of blossoming spiritual health and creativity in the face of mounting bodily wear and tear. He lived what I would call an *artful* life until its very end. Although he didn't talk about it much, I think the creative way he went about fulfilling some aspirations, long put off in the service of yet another day at the office, and the strengthening of family ties that resulted, were his way of bringing his life to spiritual peace and closure. He was in touch with his life force until his life ended.

Carpe diem is the Latin poet Virgil's phrase meaning "harvest the day." In other words, don't put off until tomorrow the things you really want to do; do them *today*. So just suppose, heaven forbid, that a doctor had just given you that same prognosis as Maurice: one more year to live. Think about all those things you've been putting off doing, those exciting things you know would really give you and your loved ones joy and fulfillment. In short, what are those things you would spend your last year on earth doing, so that at the end of it you'd have no regrets about spending too much time at the office? How would you go about making sure you hadn't missed out on anything?

To make it even easier, let's pretend there are no restrictions on this, that you have all the resources you need to fulfill every one of your dreams. Start making your list in your workbook of all the fun and deeply fulfilling things that are out there, that you never really imagined were accessible to you. It might for example be taking a cruise to Alaska or Asia or Africa. It might be learning parasailing or hang gliding or scuba diving. You might want to enroll in your local community college and learn a new language or technology, just for the sake of stretching your mind a bit. You may simply choose to deepen your personal relationships by spending more time on quiet walks and talks with friends and family.

You might yearn to spend more time with your grandchildren, like Maurice, and let them dictate each day's activities. It can be enormous fun to let children take charge of things, and not have to worry about exactly what time they get to bed. Make sure too that you include at least one art-making project on your list. Maurice took up cooking, which certainly counts as an art form. So for example does gardening, origami (the traditional Japanese art of paper-cutting), carpentry, basket-weaving, dressmaking, photography, building models of boats or cars or planes—you name it. There are countless art-making projects like these that I haven't touched on in earlier chapters.

I hope you've taken the time and made the effort to come up with a good long list of things you'd really like to pursue. Now I want you to look over your list and choose just one of these items that particularly appeals. Make it something that will engage and challenge you, but that is realistic and won't frustrate you or be incompatible with any restrictions that current illness or disability may have placed on you. I want you to make a commitment—right here and now—to actually take this one on. This will mean exploring exactly what it will take of all the external and internal resources available to you that we discussed in chapter 3. Set yourself some definite deadlines, and also tell a friend or family member, or several, of your intention, so they can help you keep your resolution to take up your new project or learn your new skill, and so enrich and deepen your life.

Spirituality and Health

The blessed reality is that most of us have many more years of healthy life still to go. Yet everyone's life does have a finite span, so this simple exercise brings your attention to bear on those activities and skills you may be missing out on. Dr. Stephen Levine (1997) has written a challenging book called just that, *A Year to Live*. He describes how he challenged himself to live for a year as though each day, each hour, each moment, were truly his last. He has developed a series of practices and meditations that force you to decide what your real priorities are, and show you to how come to a new and vibrant relationship with life in all its immediacy. In other words, how do you live every moment as though it were your last?

I said earlier that I think of the health of your spiritual self as central to all other aspects of personal and collective human health, and especially to the creative genius to which every one of us is heir. Here's another exercise to help illustrate what I mean.

Exercise: Building Blocks

Wherever you are right now, from whatever vantage point you're gazing out on the world, take a good long look around you. Notice everything that falls within your field of vision. Look at the walls of the room you're in. What are they made up of? At a guess, they're made of concrete, or bricks and mortar, covered with paint or paper. Perhaps they're reinforced with steel. Look at the chairs and bed, the cupboards and bookcases, all the other furniture in the room. What are their components? They probably contain a good amount of wood, covered with various woven fabrics, perhaps with steel and rubber attachments (handles and wheels, for instance). Each of these components, of which you see only the outward appearance, is itself made up of so many physical and chemical elements it would be impossible to number them all.

Can you see out of your window? Maybe you're several floors up. If so, think about exactly what's supporting you—more concrete and bricks and steel girders, most likely. And just think, every part of this structure was raised from the ground these several floors up by your fellow human beings. Now let yourself become aware that every such building, where you spend most of your working and playing and resting life—whether it be a private residence or a hotel or a hospital or a suite of corporate offices—is created, *made up*, block by block, beam by beam, tile by tile, by the ingenuity and imagination, coupled with the physical energy and dexterity, of individual people. And these people have worked together as an endlessly forming and reforming series of teams. Each one had all our frailty and capacity for making mistakes, but learned from these mistakes, and went on to create something seemingly *superhuman.*

If you were a geologist, or an organic chemist, or a materials engineer, you could probably describe the precise elemental composition of all these things in your range of vision pretty well. And every one of these individual elements is created originally from the tiniest invisible particles that come directly out of our glorious Earth. First it's discovered and excavated, then experimented with, then combined and synthesized, decorated and put into its final place. Actually it isn't its *final* place, because so many things are recycled today, used and reused for very many different purposes. And as I expect you learned in school, no matter is ever created or destroyed.

Contemplating the Universe

You may wonder what this preoccupation with matter and technology has to do with art-making, or with spirituality and healing. Well, allow yourself to contemplate the extraordinary and boundless creativity of whoever created all this, along with the imagination and inventiveness of the human race. Reflect for a moment: See yourself and your fellow humans, placed upon this mass of minerals and matter, and given the capacity to improve your life and health in countless ways. This evolution of the earth and all its creatures has continued over eons of time, in one long succession of God-given experiments in creativity. It's impossible to become aware of the vastness of the Earth's gifts to us—and of our own ingenuity in putting these gifts to work—without contemplating directly the source of all things, along with our relationships to each other, as the primal force that moves us to greater health and creativity.

This driving force is central to the human condition. It is the breath of our being, compelling us on our separate and collective paths through our mortal lives. The physical, mental, and social components of our health and happiness are all grounded within this spirit-filled universe. I suggest to you—whenever you're feeling a little lonely or aimless, bored or unfulfilled, or confused about the direction of your life—that you take a look at this feeling not so much as a mental or emotional problem but as a spiritual one.

Art-Making as a Spiritual Resource

Nowadays these kinds of feelings are only too frequent amongst us, to judge from what you read, hear, and see through the mass media. Human beings are becoming increasingly alienated from each other, less and less in touch with the child's sense of awe and wonder at everything around her. This is especially true in our United States, although we have the greatest riches and resources of any nation on earth.

The sad fact is that our trillion-dollar health care industry doesn't have ready answers to this spiritual illness. Health professionals have had little training in this kind of health care. Scientific advance and the specialized education of doctors aren't the answer; art is. Fortunately each one of us has access to the world's boundless riches in art through music and paintings, sculpture and poetry—all the art forms I've discussed with you. These are the readily available tools and techniques you can put to use each day of your life, to uplift and inspire you, to put the spiritual health of the young child back into you. Whatever the present condition of your body, you have great resources to call on and to be grateful for.

Story: An Attitude of Gratitude

Charlene is an eight-year-old girl with sickle cell disease. This is a lifelong and often crippling illness that affects many African Americans and other people of color. Affected people are prone to unpredictable attacks of acute pain that may last for days or weeks, and that often put them in the hospital for long periods. They're also more vulnerable to serious infections than other people, and as time goes on they often lose the full use of their arms or legs due to strokes. The working of their heart and liver and kidneys may also become strained, so they find themselves depending on a regular prescription of many drugs.

Charlene has been in our hospital four times in the past year. The last episode seemed to me the worst, mainly because it went on for so long. School was about to get out for the Christmas vacation when she was admitted. When everyone else was getting ready for the holiday celebration, Charlene was spending her time in a hospital bed hooked up to an intravenous infusion of essential fluids, coupled with a regular dose of morphine for her persistent back and leg pain.

What inspired me was her never-failing attitude of acceptance and abundant gratitude for her blessings. Every day I'd go into her room and perch on the end of her bed. (I did this gingerly because the pressure of a weight on her blankets could add to her pain.) I'd ask her how she was feeling. Never a day went by that she didn't answer: "I'm better today." If I pressed her a little more, she'd say that, yes, her appetite was a bit better, that she'd managed some grits for breakfast, or that it had been a bit easier getting to the bathroom that morning. And each day she'd let us try cutting down on the amount of her pain meds, so she could be more wakeful and less dependent on others for help. But time and again it became clear that it was still too early to do so.

I don't know which came first, Charlene's courageous "attitude of gratitude," or the loving care toward her of her family. Never a day passed that there wasn't at least one family member with her. Both sets of grandparents lived out of state, but they all found time to visit and spend time with their granddaughter, while giving her parents a break, since both of them had jobs they needed to hold down. Almost every afternoon Charlene's mother would bring her healthy brother and sister to see her, complete with toys and games from home. On the last day of school, her teacher showed up, having given three of Charlene's best friends a ride so they could visit too. While the staff were all deeply appreciative of this support from family and friends, for me it seemed it was Charlene's grace-filled attitude toward her illness that inspired everyone around her.

Exercise: Your Extended Family

So now I want you to create a picture of your own extended family. To do this you'll need a blank sheet of your workbook or sketchbook, together with crayons or colored pencils.

Start off by drawing as big a circle as your page will contain (like you did for your personal mandala). Now put yourself in the middle of the circle, like the bull's-eye at the center of a dartboard. You can represent yourself by a stick figure or simply with a smiley face, or you may want to depict yourself in detailed and glorious Technicolor. Now start filling in the remaining space with other people in your life. Begin with your *inner circle*—those closest to you. They're going to form a tight circle around you. Most people have at least half a dozen folks who are close to them through family ties or friendship. Let these people—or pets—surround you in a loving and supportive way, even if for some reason you aren't feeling very close to one or another of them right now. Color them different colors for added interest, as your muse inspires you. Represent each one with whatever size and shape you feel moved to. Don't forget to add their names, because you're going to end up with a sizable collection of your extended family.

Now start gradually moving outwards. Let your mind extend to other current friends and family, so they complete your second circle, again in multiple shapes and sizes and colors as you feel inclined. Put their names in too. Now for your third circle, surrounding the last one, think about others who have peopled your life at earlier times. These might be grandparents, uncles and aunts, for example, who maybe aren't living anymore. Or perhaps friends will come to mind who've moved on, so you're no longer in touch, but of whom you still have fond memories. Think of all those friends and neighbors from towns you've lived in at other times of your life. Include girl-friends and boyfriends too—and perhaps your very first love. And don't forget those teachers you had in the various schools you attended. Can you remember their names?

You should by now be nearing the outer edges of your circle. Most people have many dozens of little portraits by now, going back over the years of their lives. Take a few more minutes to add any others that come into your mind. How about some pets: dogs and cats or a hamster or gerbil or two? Or even a favorite tree from your childhood? You may well want to represent them with animal likenesses or symbols. Can you remember all their names and characteristics, and what on earth happened to them?

Most people who do this exercise are astonished when they come to fully realize the size and number of the extended family they've accumulated over their lifetimes. It can get to feel pretty cozy nestling in the middle of all these human and other beings who've shared your life, many for considerable periods. Take a look at these figures or faces looking up at you. There's really no reason to ever feel lonely or lost again.

Loss

This leads on to another aspect of illness and disability I want to talk with you about—one for which art-making can be an especially helpful tool. I'm referring to all the *losses* you've experienced in your life, which are an unavoidable part of the human condition.

Some such losses are quite trivial, or even funny, particularly when seen from the vantage point of months or years later. Smaller losses may even serve to divert you from the threat of a larger, more serious one. I remember losing a camera when my canoe capsized far from anywhere, way down upon the Suwannee River, with the water running almost at flood tide. My friend and I were lucky to get out alive that day. All I could talk about, as we dried ourselves off on the mosquito-infested river bank and tried to get help finding our way back to civilization, was my poor little camera, sunk to the bottom of the river complete with an almost finished roll of film.

Most people would say that the greatest loss any human being sustains is loss of life, first the lives of those close to them and ultimately their own. While this is often the case, it isn't invariably so. There are many smaller losses in life that may be just as painful and evoke just as much physical, emotional, and spiritual suffering. If you or a loved one are affected by a serious illness or disability, you have every reason to know what I mean. After all, the dying process may be extremely painful, but death itself isn't at all, as far as we know. In fact, it's very often blessed as being the final end to physical and other forms of pain for the dying person. This is not to diminish the often deep and prolonged bereavement of those left behind.

The Life Cycle of Grief

The painful feelings a serious loss evokes in a person, and those close to them, are as much spiritual as emotional and physical. These reactions are summed up in the one word *grief*, which comes from the Latin word *gravitas*, meaning "weight" or "burden." Loss weighs down your spirit, so that nothing seems worthwhile anymore. Life has ceased to be fun. The first time a child loses a pet—maybe just a tadpole from a jar or a beetle from a matchbox—not only creates the anguish of realizing they'll never see their friend again, it also leads to that unanswerable question, "Why?" It awakens the child to the transitory nature of all human life. Many parents and teachers find that the loss of pets is a helpful doorway to discussions of such larger issues with their children. Perhaps you've found this too.

When a child gets a bit older, she starts to encounter other experiences of loss, as when a young boy finds he's considered too old to get into bed with his parents for a snuggle, or a little girl is told she can't share the nighttime bath with her big brother anymore. Suddenly a second-grader's best friend takes up with someone else in school. Or a young boy doesn't make it onto the softball or soccer team, or a girl no longer makes it to the top grades when she moves up a class. Every child loses treasured possessions, through carelessness or in the move to a new house, through theft or by simple wear and tear. A teenager discovers the heartbreak of his first lost love affair, and soon after this the loss of safety of hearth and home when he goes away to college.

These are the beginnings, the preparation for a lifetime of losses we all experience. Illness and disability are examples of losses adults encounter as they age, with their accompanying reduction in physical fitness and independence. These losses—call them *little deaths*—can be thought of as a lifetime's preparation for the final loss of mortal life.

Art-Making as an Antidote to Grief

The grief of loss and bereavement, then, is part of our lives from beginning to end. This isn't to say that life isn't full of joy too. It's simply in the nature of things that to know ecstasy and deep fulfillment you must also experience your share of suffering, disappointment, and frustration. But what most of us aren't taught in our lives is how to deal with grief and learn from it.

From reading this far you'll have discovered that much of the art-making I've been teaching you has been used in many cultures for healing purposes from way back in prehistory. As a society we're only just coming back to this realization, and starting to put art to work once more for our greater health. Several of the stories you've heard have to do directly with recovery from the grieving process. Look at the stories of Danny and Rose in chapter 1, Julie in chapter 5, and Maurice in the current chapter, as examples of people turning to art under the immediate threat of loss of life. Marie in chapter 2 turned the falling of her beautiful hair into a direct expression of her creativity. Carl in chapter 3 and Brenda in chapter 4 put art to work to give them back a sense of control over their lives in a world that seemed set on taking it away from them.

Lots of examples of art being used for this purpose have been reported in medical and other health care journals. The music therapist and founder of the Chalice of Repose project, Therese Schroeder-Sheker (1994), has shown the benefits of harp and vocal music for giving back comfort and dignity to dying persons, and assisting the grieving process of their families. Give me harp music at my bedside when my time comes. Art therapist Cathy Malchiodi has edited a book, *Medical Art Therapy with Adults* (1999), capturing in one place many studies of the visual arts as comfort and inspiration at times of grief or impending bereavement. I discussed in chapter 5 Dr. Pennebaker's studies showing the value of creative writing to help resolve past traumas that are still causing grief and emotional distress. Lastly, Dr. Sandra Bertman has edited a book, *Grief and the Healing Arts* (1999), devoted entirely to grief work through the creative arts. Although directed primarily at caregivers and therapists, it's a valuable resource for laypeople too in how pictures and poems, songs and films, can come to your service when you're at a loss for words to express painful or confusing feelings.

Stories: Artists Using Art to Heal Themselves

I've mentioned several times the program I helped create at my hospital called Arts in Medicine. Many of the artists and their students have come to the work as a result of personal discoveries of the healing power of their art-making.

Our codirector, Mary Rockwood-Lane, who created the artists-in-residence program, came to it as a nurse and a painter at a time when she was herself very ill, and beginning to despair that she would ever find a way out of her emotional pain and grief. She speaks in the introductory chapter of the book *Creative Healing* (1998, p. 22), which she co-wrote with physician and artist Michael Samuels, about how throwing herself into her creative work gave her immediate and powerful benefits. "I needed my whole life enmeshed in it because that was how I was involved with my sickness. Creative healing transformed my life. I pulled it out of myself and healed myself. . . . My illness was so overwhelming I needed to live my healing all the time. . . . I could always be there for myself."

Our dancer-in-residence, Jill Sonke-Henderson, tells a similar story in *Creative Healing* of how the healing power of dance came to her during a serious illness that kept her confined to bed as a young adult. She was just starting out in her career as a professional dancer when a serious infection overtook her, and she was in too much pain to move. She used visualization while listening to music on the radio in bed, and danced all day inside her body. "I could feel that energy swirling, and it felt really alive and wonderful. . . . It was like being out of my body, even though I was just lying there. . . . I think it helped the healing in that the energy was moving inside me, causing flow, instead of me just feeling that nothing was happening" (p. 198). It was this experience that led Jill to link her training as a dancer to working with hospital patients and teaching them how dance and movement could help in their healing. In talking about the process, she puts it this way: "You find that place that is just free. Freedom, just space—no time—it's just space and it's just energy and then you ride it. . . ."

Michael Samuels, Mary's coauthor, tells the story of journaling when his wife was going through a marrow transplant to try to cure her of advanced breast cancer. "I wrote a journal about the experience, and that probably saved my life then. . . . For reasons I didn't know, I decided to bring a laptop into her room and write each day. . . . Instead of being sad or being a crisis report, my journal became deeply spiritual. It became a story of bravery and of Nancy as my teacher" (53). As a result of this urge to create in the face of crisis, Michael's inner artist emerged, letting him see his wife and himself, and what was happening to them both, in a way that was sustaining, not depressing.

My own epiphany about art and healing happened ten years ago. I had already been a pediatrician caring for children with cancer and their families for twenty years, always finding it deeply fulfilling work. There'd been a huge improvement in treatment over this time, such that well over half these young people with once uniformly fatal illness were growing to adulthood free of cancer. Many were having healthy children of their own. And they had always inspired me with their courage and resilience in the face of such life challenges. I deeply loved the close relationships we could build between us.

But I became more and more aware that the work was very taxing to staff morale, and that many doctors and nurses were feeling the burden of caring for patients with such serious illness. I'd started to write a journal of my experiences, which had helped me be less the doctor-scientist and more the gatherer of stories of courage and inspiration. This led me to poetry. I started to create poems out of these stories, and I published them in medical journals. I've written more about this in an article on the connection between poetry and my work with these children (Graham-Pole 1996).

After a reading at the annual conference of poetry therapists, one of the audience members said she'd enjoyed my poems, but could I bring a little more lightness to bear on my subject matter? Did everything have to be so gloomy? It was then that it struck me: The whole of medicine had become such a *serious business*. It wasn't just those who were looking after children with cancer but the whole of the health profession that seemed to have ceased to have fun anymore. By chance I ran into two friends at work, Mary Clark, a recreational therapist, and Jane Cheney, an occupational therapist, who'd started to explore ways in which they could use more motivational humor with their clients. We decided to offer humor workshops to staff as well as patients as a way to lighten up the heavy atmosphere we were encountering.

This proved more successful than we'd ever expected. In no time we found ourselves doing an end-of-year program for the hospital's administrators, at a time when morale was at low ebb, thanks to the hospital's shrinking budget and a lot of staff layoffs. From that point we started to work regularly with nurses and doctors, medical technologists and dietitians, as well as groups of patients and their families, always using humor and laughter as a key to unlock feelings of tension and distress. Since that time, "playshops" have become a regular part of my work as a doctor. Together with poetry, they've played a huge part in restoring creativity and inspiration to my daily life.

Exercise: Healing Wounds

So now you have the opportunity to practice your artist's insights and skills, to see if they can be helpful to you in dealing with an incompletely resolved loss.

Think about something that is currently causing you grief. It might not spring immediately to mind, so give yourself a little time to let it surface. Sometimes we drift along through life without realizing we're being increasingly weighed down by past griefs and traumas—like a gunnysack of stuff that drags on the floor behind us and gets caught in elevator doors. You might alight on a recent happening, for example impaired physical ability through illness or injury. An older man I know chose the issue of the diminishing force of his urine stream caused by prostate enlargement. You might focus on the loss of your ability to remember names and dates, or to think of things quickly during a conversation. It might be the loss of a loved one, either recently or in the more distant past; this is something that has happened to all of us. Old losses—even from childhood—can linger for years, or lifetimes, and have serious long-term effects on your overall health.

Once you have something in mind, you're going to choose your art form. Let me remind you of a few ways you've learned to express your feelings and thoughts in the last few chapters. You've found, I hope, that capturing images in your mind and on paper can have great healing effects. You've learned to create a mandala, and to use twelve-speed writing for problem-solving. You've practiced splitting story-time with a close friend or family member, and you've put the art of poetry to work. You've experienced the healing balm of reading yourself a cozy childhood story before sleep, or better still being read to. You've tried your hand at singing funny songs, even or especially when you don't feel at all like doing so. And you've strutted your stuff in many different ways as dancer and actor and comic, learning how each of these art forms can give you meaning and insight, even in the face of severe suffering. You've learned how each can have lasting healing effects on your body, mind, and spirit.

Give yourself about twenty minutes initially, although you may well find that you get into a project that will take longer, or will require several sessions. As you've discovered, most exercises in this book are adaptable to this format. I remember a group of women with breast cancer who started work on a quilt, with the purpose of expressing their personal and collective stories about the losses they'd suffered—not least the loss of either one or both breasts. They knew from the outset that their project was a long-term one that wasn't going to get done in a single session.

It's again ideal for you to work with a partner, or several, on this exercise, taking it in turns to do your wound-healing through art-making. This way the others can serve as supportive audience, or even as coaches. You may each want to work simultaneously, then come back together to share your creations, and how they've been helpful or not, as the case may be. It's fine too to do this exercise alone, but I can't stress enough the value of sharing your stories of loss and its accompanying grief with others. Remember that art-making, in this book anyway, is a communal activity.

Love: The Healing Force

Which brings me to the final topic of this chapter: love. I've urged you throughout to approach any illness or disability you or a loved one may have as a chance to expand your awareness of things in the world, and to discover artful ways to enhance your whole health in the face of whatever adversity affects you. This is a tall order. It may be tempting on many days to roll over and succumb to whatever affliction has struck, and ask no questions. It may seem much easier to take whatever medicine gives you temporary physical relief, in whatever quantity you need it. Hence the vital importance to you of building your support system, and of having allies to help you on every step of the way.

Cardiologist Dean Ornish said in his book *Love and Survival* (1998, p. 2) that, of all the medicines we human beings have available to us to heal ourselves and others, love is the single most potent. He writes: "I am not aware of any other factor in medicine that has a greater impact on our survival than the healing power of love and intimacy. Not diet, not smoking, not exercise, not stress, not genetics, not drugs, not surgery." Both men and women are at less risk of severe heart disease if they have deep emotional relationships with others. Studies of elders have shown that you can limit the effects of aging even more by what you contribute to your social support network than what you get back.

However, the most powerful aspect of love is its two-way nature: We are, at one time or another—hopefully all the time—loved right back by friends and family, by those we come to help, by lovers, and of course by God. Paradoxically, though, the best kind of love is that which is unconditional and asks nothing in return. So what Dr. Ornish and others who have studied the healing effects of close relationships are saying is that the more we share unconditional love with others, the better will be our overall wellness, personally and collectively. I introduced you to some of these studies in the first chapter. We now know that whether you have some serious condition like heart disease or cancer or AIDS, or you're just getting older and less independent than you used to be, the close companionship of others can be lifesaving.

Two classic books on the art of loving, C. S. Lewis's *The Four Loves* (1960) and Erich Fromm's *The Art of Loving* (1957), pinpoint the same basic categories of love: affection, friendship, erotic love, and the love of God. I suspect that every one of us has experienced each of these in plentiful measure at some point in our lives. Each seems instinctive. We all feel loving affection for our family members and close friends. We experience a loving feeling toward those in need whom we're able to help in some way. I hope every one of you has enjoyed the ecstasy of romantic love toward a spouse or a sweetheart. And the love that transcends earthly love is that which many, perhaps most, humans come to feel for their creator.

Exercise: A Gift of Art

As a final exercise in this chapter, I invite you to create a gift of art to someone for whom you feel love or affection. As we've seen, this offers more than just the warm glow you feel inside from gift-giving. Such a tangible expression of your feelings for someone close to you, or who has been of service to you, can have real health-giving benefits.

First, spend some time thinking about who you would like to give your work of art to. It might of course be your spouse or a close family member, especially if you have recently had to depend on them more than you would wish. The same goes for a close friend or someone in your support group of whom you've grown fond. It might be a caregiver you've come to know well, perhaps your doctor or a favorite nurse. Or it might be someone you don't know so well, but who seems to have more troubles to deal with than you, and is in need of a show of affection. You may want to make a special gift for your creator, like the little boy spied going into a church and laying his baseball mitt on the altar as his personal gift to God.

Once again I'm going to encourage you to choose the kind of art you create for your chosen one. Start by going back over your workbook and sketchbook, and any other materials you've gathered. You may have something you've been treasuring—shells or bits of ornamental glass or beads you can work into a piece of jewelry. There may be some visual art you want to offer that you're especially pleased with. You may want to create something similar again, using it as inspiration to make another original work. Look at the writing you've done. Perhaps you have a few lines of poetry, a letter, or other creative writing that you're proud of, or that you can use as a stepping-off point for something new. You may have put the words of a simple song down on paper, and now you want to brush it up for your chosen one. Perhaps you've become courageous with dancing and feel up to choreographing a simple dance as a love offering.

As I hope you've accepted by now, it isn't the technical brilliance of the artwork that matters. What counts is that it has some vital meaning for you. As you picture your spouse or friend, your caregiver or the one you've decided needs a little loving attention, give thought to what would fit them well and have special significance. What do you know about them? What have they meant to you? Why did you pick them out especially? Some of the loveliest gifts I've ever received are simple letters of gratitude that say something about me that the person has noticed or is fond of.

Once you've decided what you're going to give, and have worked on it for as long as you need to, then it's important to make a little ceremony of the gift-giving. You may want to have a few others present, to whom it will have significance. You might for example choose an anniversary of some kind, or the day of your going home if you've selected a caregiver. Be sure to prepare a little speech to go with your gift. Let them know what this gift especially means to you.

Take time to notice how you feel in creating this personal symbol of love for another human being. It's likely to be very gratifying. Write a few lines in your workbook or journal to mark the event and its significance for you. How wonderful to have used art as an expression of your appreciation, compassion, and love.

10

Bringing It All Together

Do it now; there may be a law against it tomorrow.

—Laurence Peter

What Have You Learned?

In this final chapter, it's time to take stock. We've kept each other company on a long journey of discovery, or rather of rediscovery. I've offered you a lot of challenges. I've asked you on many occasions to put aside your doubts and inhibitions, your weariness and weaknesses, your concerns about what others might think of you. Some, perhaps much, of what I've asked of you may seem strange or downright silly. You may not have felt immediate benefits. Perhaps you even found yourself feeling worse at first, as half-buried memories have surfaced to sadden or worry you once more. New challenges may perhaps have caused you frustration or anger.

But I hope that alongside any negative experiences, you've allowed yourself an equal dose of pride in your accomplishments. I also hope you've offered yourself a loving spoonful of self-forgiveness, especially if you feel you've come up short in your efforts to recreate your illness or disability through the tools of art-making. I've said often in this book that your greatest enemy is your own doubt in yourself.

Story: A Thriver Not a Survivor

I have a friend and colleague, Hedi Schleiffer, who is well known as a psychotherapist and—with her husband Yumi—a workshop presenter on many aspects of health and relationship all around the world. About three years ago she was diagnosed with breast cancer. She took the opportunity this life-challenging illness presented to, as she put it, "embrace cancer with passion." This was the passion of one who saw herself as tougher and smarter than it was. She saw her cancer (always with a small "c," she insists) not as an enemy, but as a teacher. However, she was not about to let it push her around, like some teachers are inclined to. She was going to show this cancer just who it was messing with here. She built herself a network of supportive friends, family, and hospital staff: "The Boob Brigade," she called them, all "rallying around the boob." She recommends that everyone with such a serious illness make up a new name for it. She called her own cancer her "cellular challenge."

Hedi's back to full and vibrant health once more, but she takes strong exception to the phrase you've probably heard often: cancer survivor. "I'm not a cancer survivor," she says, "I'm a thriver. Saying I'm a survivor makes me feel like I'll be hanging onto some weighty burden for the rest of my life—a life sentence that I'm stuck with. I'm not 'a cancer survivor,' I'm Hedi Schleiffer—and proud of it!"

Her message is to think of health, not illness, and to see anything that has happened to you in the past—no matter how traumatic—as just an interesting historical fact of yesteryear, now over and done with for good. "Grab life with passion, embrace it with reckless abandon!" she declares.

Exercise: Self-Affirmations

Hedi is an inspiring example of someone who approached her illness from a place of centeredness and self-esteem. She knew her worth, and had no trouble affirming it. She's another of those people I call an *artist in life*. So here's an exercise in giving yourself the same kind of congratulatory pat on the back. You're going to practice *affirmations*. Webster's defines *affirmation* as a solemn and positive declaration of something you know to be true. Making declarations about your true self will help you take a final, firm stand against any lingering self-doubt.

If there were any people in your early life who caused you to doubt yourself because of their critical judgment, or because of the poor grades they handed you, try this affirmation out loud right now: "Ah, if only (my dad or Miss so-and-so my third-grade teacher, or my big sister Susan, or whoever) could see me now, how proud they'd be at how well I've turned out!" A simpler version, ideal for your very first glimpse of yourself in the mirror in the morning, is to take a firm, upright stance, puff yourself up a bit, put a big grin on your face, and declare out loud: "Wow, just look at me, world—some hot potato!"

Here's another affirmation, an extension of the exercise "Taking Pride" that you did with a partner in chapter 3. Whenever anyone pays you a compliment, however minor, like for example: "Your hair looks nice today," or "What a great job you've done on this room," try responding quick as a flash—before any self-put-downs can set in—"Thanks for noticing!" No one will ever take you for a show-off, because this is a nice funny rejoinder. But it does the trick of bolstering your self-esteem once more. If you want to keep the joke going a bit longer, follow up with: "Hey, tell me more. I've got plenty of time. So you like my hair, huh? So what else looks good about me? I want all the details now!"

This is a pretty irresistible line, so practice and use it lots, especially with all your artworks. "So you like my work, huh? Well, just how good is it—this picture (or poem, or song, or dance, or whatever)? No hurry, take your time telling me all the good stuff."

Taking Stock

Let's summarize all you've covered in this book. I haven't asked you to proceed in an orderly or disciplined fashion, because art wasn't meant to go in a straight line. But I hope by now you've convinced yourself—with a little help from me—that making art can give your health and well-being a huge shot in the arm. Through these pages you've had a chance to get to know a lot of people and hear their stories. I've tried to offer you examples of folks I've known who've used art in its many forms to help themselves when life had dealt them a hard blow and they were up against it. I hope they've inspired you.

I've taught you about the ancient history of art for health, and how hospitals and other places of health care are beginning to bring art-making once more into the forefront, with the encouragement of people like you and me. You've learned of the connection between symptoms and symbols—how art can help you make sense of an illness and find new meaning in it. I've stressed the value of telling your story in different ways, as well as listening to those of others. We are all of us simply the stories of our lives.

Through storytelling and art-making I hope you've become a *groupie*, building a support group for yourself that will nurture you, no matter what. I trust you've made a new friend of your doctor and other caregivers, and felt the power of taking charge of your circumstances with some of the resources I've offered you. I trust you've got a clearer grasp on whatever health issues are affecting you, and the vital part you can play in helping yourself, not leaving it to others to take charge and issue you doctor's orders.

Perhaps during the course of your reading you've become an inspired visualizer, a mindful meditator, a jotter and journal writer, a dedicated doodler, a pretty painter and poet, a sweet singer and dancer. You've tapped, I'm sure, into resources both inner and outer that you had been hitherto unaware of. You've reclaimed your *space*, whatever your outward restrictions may be, establishing a studio-retreat for yourself. Within this space, you've made room for displaying your works of art, making them readily accessible to you. You've made it easy for yourself to cherish them and pore over them, to modify and extend them. You've let yourself share them often with others, whenever the need and opportunity has arisen.

You've become, I know, fully aware once more of the happy and playful young child still alive and kicking inside you, no matter what your age or degree of disability may be. This is the child who giggles and chortles at next to nothing, sees the funny side of just about anything, and finds any number of ways to solve a problem or get a thing done. This is the child who bounces back from affliction with resilience and creativity, after shedding a few well-earned and healthy tears, or perhaps staging a tantrum or two—in an appropriate setting. And as a child of God once more, I fully expect you've re-learned the universal message of illness and of disability: the blessed chance it affords you to *slow down*.

Because illness is one thing that forces you to ease up on your hectic pace, smell not just the roses but every good aroma to be sniffed, relish the sight of nature, the sound of music, and the taste of food. It especially gives you permission to feel once more, in your hands and ears, on your lips and feet, the new-but-old familiarity of those implements of art-making I've reintroduced you to.

In claiming art as friend and supporter once more, I dearly hope you've also come to experience the *life force*, that authentic and undying spirit within you. I trust you've learned to fill your lungs and heart with its inspiration, and to celebrate life again, no matter what may be your infirmity or limitation. I fully anticipate you've learned the essential art of *carpe diem*—of living each God-given moment as though it were your last. I hope you are hearkening to the truth of the old saying: "Life is so short we should move very slowly."

So are you doing so right now? Are you moving slowly, letting yourself fully celebrate your love of life, of every person in your life, and of your very own self? I very much hope so.

Story: The Gift of Sight

A woman I'll call Margaret has been a patient at our hospital for several reasons. She's in her late sixties, and has had diabetes since she was a child. Recently it had been causing her all kinds of complications, the way diabetes can do. She'd had difficulty walking, her heart was feeling the strain, and, worst of all, she was progressively losing her eyesight.

I'd gotten to know her pretty well, because she volunteered with us as an artist. She would show up each week regular as clockwork on the heart transplant unit. Having had such a lot of personal experience of illness, but never having let herself be discouraged or immobilized by it, she quickly endeared herself to patients young and old. Because her sight was failing, she could no longer produce the lovely watercolors that had been her special forte, so she simply switched over to writing short stories about her many experiences of the hospital and health care folks.

The nature of a heart transplant unit is that the patients mostly have severe and intractable heart conditions that can only be helped substantially by the gift of a new heart. Since there's a strictly limited number of suitable hearts available, and always a long waiting list, many spend weeks and months on the cardiac unit. They get to know each other well; it's a ready-made support group. Margaret would come every Thursday afternoon to paint T-shirts or make simple jewelry with the patients. As this became more difficult, she switched over to reading one of her stories—full of wry humor and color. Finally she needed a wheelchair, and couldn't see well enough to read them herself. But she'd still find one of us to get her there, and have people take it in turns to read her stories.

Margaret has never lost her resilience, her creativity, or her joy in the company of others who are sharing equal or greater burdens of illness. Although she can see very little nowadays, she still brings a precious gift of vision to her friends and loved ones: the vision of heart and spirit that links us all. And she continues to be grateful for every day granted to her.

Exercise: Thankfulness

I invite you to spend a few minutes thinking about your current situation, but strictly from the viewpoint of giving thanks.

It's often easier to do this exercise with a friend, but it's by no means essential. Just make yourself comfy, take out your workbook, and start making a list of all the things in your life that you have to be thankful for. (Remember that the French word for "wound" is *blessure*, or blessing.) The only rule of this exercise is that you don't include anything you cannot turn into some kind of blessing.

It may help you if you go back to those inner resources you took a look at in chapter 3. I'm specifically talking about being mindful of your surroundings, and of the present moment, so as to increase your emotional self-awareness. Try taking stock of your immediate environment, taking in everything you see around you. If you're in a hospital room where you've been for some time, you may become aware of all the cards and other symbols of well-wishing you've accumulated. Or try gazing out of your window at the sunshine or rain in the trees, and be simply thankful for all the beauty of our earth that is still there for you to enjoy.

Become aware too of your body, and how it's still functioning remarkably well, keeping you shuffling, or even scooting through each day—even if there are parts of it that could use a bit of oiling or a new coat of paint. How are your taste buds? Are you still able to enjoy many of the delights of good cooking? If you're getting on in years, perhaps you've still got the ability to get around without help, or the capacity for smelling flowers, seeing a rainbow, or hearing beautiful music. Do you still have a good, strong grip in your hands, or a fine head of hair? Be grateful, and add it to your list.

I want you to keep going until you've listed at least twenty items you're grateful for in this life. As you can see, they don't have to be very grand or complex things. One of the gifts of age, for example, is very often the growth of family—the birth of grandchildren or great-nephews and great-nieces. Even if you don't get to see them often, what a wonderful gift to have young ones in your family. If you're still young yourself, you may want to dwell on all the infinite possibilities that await you, fantasizing about how things may well turn out just the way you want them.

Take no more than ten minutes to jot down all the things you can think of that you're grateful for. You may well want to keep going, or just to keep this list handy for adding to. My experience is that whenever things don't seem to be going too well, a quick review of all the things I have to be thankful for will always lift my spirits.

Art Is Multimedia

One of the things you may have noticed is that at no time have I suggested to you that one form of artwork is best for one condition or illness or disability, and another type of art-making for something quite different. When we started the arts program at our hospital ten years ago, we found artists to help us who were mostly experienced and skilled at one art form. It didn't take us long to discover that it worked best if the artists laid aside all their learned notions, and simply brought with them their creativity and an open mind. What happened was that Jill, our dancer, started trying her hand at poetry, while Ellie, our writer and storyteller, found herself as often as not with a paintbrush in her hands. The great thing about this was that it helped level the playing field, as the patients and their families realized that these professional artists were venturing into new territory alongside them.

It comes back to something I've told you pretty often in various ways: that it isn't about how good you are as an artist, but about taking your courage and your curiosity on a journey of exploration. You absolutely do not have to have special ability to make art. All you need is a spirit of adventure and fun, and the belief that your creative intelligence is always there, waiting patiently to serve you and to do you good. It's true that most of the evidence I've mentioned is focused on one art form being tried with a given group of patients with similar conditions. But I am of the strong belief that if you express your thoughts and feelings through creative self-expression, it doesn't matter what medium you work in. Writing or painting or working with clay, singing or enjoying creative games or dancing or play-acting—they're all after the same instinctive goal. Art-making is another way of knowing yourself, of giving yourself permission, of working out your problems, of taking creative charge of your life. In learning these new-but-old skills, you've opened the doors wide to greater self-fulfillment.

Exercise: Mixing and Matching

So here's an exercise in playing your many attempts at art-making off against each other.

I want you to collect all your pieces together—workbook, journal, artwork, painted clothing, homemade jewelry, mandalas, songs, poems, collages—no matter what. There may be among them several works of art that feel unfinished to you, or are simply scribblings or fragments. That's just fine. Hopefully you have a real diversity of art-making before you. The only thing they have in common is their creator.

The purpose of this is to reexplore how each one reflects a part of you. Then I'll invite you to mix and match them, to see what such a juxtaposition brings up. Take, for example, the personal mandala you created in chapter 4. You made a big circle and put yourself inside it, as a crayon stick-figure or a balloon. Then you embellished it with several aspects of yourself: your body, mind, and spirit, as well as your relationships with others and with your environment. It was an exercise in imagination of yourself and your health. Have you taken it out and looked at it lately? What does it have to say to you today? Is there anything you want to add to it? Or would you like to do a new version of it, to reflect where you've come from since then?

Now see if your personal mandala—an example of visual art at work—suggests to you any other form of art other than drawing with crayons. Are there some words, perhaps a short poem that you'd like to write about it? Perhaps you could turn these words of yours into a song. Take a good look at whatever you've produced, then close your eyes and start to move your body in dance. Remember that for dancing it's not important if you're in bed, you just move in rhythm whatever parts of your body you can, in any way you feel moved to. You might try adding your song to your dance, as a kind of hymn of celebration to yourself.

Now how about the poem you wrote in chapter 5? You started with just three or four words on each of ten lines, all with a different subject. Then you chose one line at random that offered itself to you, and you created a poem out of that moment of your day. Do you remember? Looking back on it today, what are the images that come to you? I invite you to draw with your chalks or pastels or colored pencils those images, as a complement to your poem—perhaps the first poem you'd written for years.

When you've done that, take a good look at this new creation. Then close your eyes and once more offer up a song and dance that seems to go with it. You may want to jot down the words to your song. Is it a sad song or a joyful one? Does it have a fast or slow tempo? How about the rhythm of your body? Do you feel moved toward a rapid jerky rhythm—or a slow, sinuous one? After a few minutes, open your eyes once more and take another look at all your treasures. Is there any other piece of artwork that seems to be asking to be included in this multimedia celebration?

Do you recall some of the wacky games I urged you to try in chapter 8? You learned about collecting toys and silly props, and about galumphing—doing everyday, routine things in unusual and deliberately harder ways. How about trying some of these once more, and then drawing a picture or composing a little song about your silly self? You might like to throw in some of those tongue-twisting medical phrases that I hope you made up. . . .

You can do this kind of multimedia exercise with any of the individual exercises you've completed in this book. As you go through the process, take note of what seems easiest and what is harder. Some ways of making art will come more naturally to you than others, but all of them can be helpful and health-enhancing.

Other Ways of Making Art

In making art, we as human beings are only limited by our creativity, and that knows absolutely no limits! There are many forms of art-making I haven't even touched on in this book. I'll do so briefly now.

Cooking

Take, for example, the culinary arts—the delight of cooking. There are few things more expressive than this of your innate creativity. Good food deliciously prepared for your table appeals to so many of your senses: sight and smell and touch and taste. It's endlessly creative, and it's a time-honored way to spend time with your loved ones. If you have the chance to prepare food for a meal at your own whim and your own pace—cutting and stirring and grinding and kneading—without it being an obligation as the meal provider of the household, it can be an endlessly fulfilling activity.

You've probably heard that phrase "comfort food." At times of stress or loneliness, I've sometimes found myself very comforted by simple foods that my mom used to prepare for me as a child. I think for example of boiled eggs and fingers of toast, steaming hot oatmeal with treacle, and loaves of gingerbread. What are your lifelong favorites? Perhaps they may not be considered health foods in today's diet-conscious world, but why not indulge yourself in a few comfort foods when you feel the yen?

Of course many light and simple food combinations are health-promoting by their very nature. Just let your mind dwell for a moment on all the earth's produce that you've relished over the course of your lifetime: the fresh vegetables and fruits, the nuts and grains, the meat and fish, the legumes and dairy products. Perhaps your health or your lifestyle restricts you from eating some of these things, but I know of very few people—except right after an operation—whose diet is such that they can't enjoy any of the delights of eating.

Gardening

This brings us to the endlessly creative art of gardening—of - cultivating all manner of living things in the soil. One of the greatest deprivations of being in a hospital for any length of time is that it takes you away from direct contact with the earth and living things. Plants, whether wild or cultivated, are lasting sources of both beauty and value. Not only does every plant beautify our surroundings, it also serves animals and countless smaller beings as a source of habitat and nourishment. And, like food, plants satisfy several of our special senses simultaneously: sight and touch and smell and taste.

If you don't have access to a garden, or you don't have the ability to get down in your flower beds to plant and weed, you can satisfy your need to be surrounded by flowers and greenery by cultivating indoor plants. Regardless of how limited the space around you is, you can use indoor plants to enrich your surroundings and to calm and uplift you during the turmoil of everyday life. I know folks who make an art of weeding, working on a small plot of land and priding themselves in keeping it completely clear of a single weed, so as to create a beautiful place for new plants.

And plants have needs of their own. I think you'll have grasped by now that there's as much joy to be derived from serving others through your art-making as nurturing yourself with art. A few plants growing quietly and unobtrusively around you will soon come to be your friends, looking to you for care and understanding, while offering you in return their silent and loving attention.

You may find questions raised about bringing plants into hospitals or other places of health care, but as with many other areas, the rules are getting relaxed a lot, and a few small house plants are unlikely to pose a problem. Doctors and hospital administrators are recognizing that any possible hazard from live plants is probably well outweighed by their value as a source of nurturance and solace to the patients in their care.

So try getting your hands into some handfuls of growing things. You don't have to be an expert; just allow yourself to feel the very physical joy of this experience, one that can ground you and calm you whenever things seem to be getting a bit out of control. This isn't a book of horticulture, though, any more than it's a cookbook, so I'm not going to get into details about different plants and their habits and needs here. There are plenty of very user-friendly books written by experts. Suffice to say that you can buy many indoor plants—both of the flowering variety and those with decorative foliage—at a good-sized grocery store.

Some of my favorites—both for their beauty and their forgiving hardiness—are flowers such as cyclamen, poinsettia, amaryllis, and hyacinth in the winter; and plants with variegate green foliage such as philodendron, maidenhair fern, grape ivy, and the Brazilian prayer plant. All these plants need is a little attention to watering and feeding, light and temperature—and most of them come with these instructions. It does help though to know what direction your window faces, and what control you have over the temperature of the room.

Photography and Films

Then there's photography and film. There are lots of good movies out there today, concerned with all aspects of your physical, emotional, and spiritual health. (And the ready availability of VCRs is a great help as far as accessibility goes.) Watching a movie is a perfect way to spend time together companionably with family members or friends. It's also an excellent resource for sharing the wide range of human experience, from inspiration and comedy to triumph over tragedy. Don't we all relish the idea of going to the movies for a good laugh and a good cry? That was certainly one of the reasons for the success of the film of Patch Adams' life—it got you both laughing and crying in plenty.

Earlier I mentioned a program I call Medical Student Buddies at my hospital. It brings new students into direct contact with patients and their families as friends, or extended family members, rather than as part of the health care team. The students benefit by seeing serious illness from the viewpoint of the patient, while the patient gets an extra source of support beyond immediate family members, who may be as distressed by the illness as the patients themselves. Movies are a favorite communal activity for these buddies, and the students have learned the favorites: the ones that evoke the liveliest and perhaps most intimate discussions about health and illness, and even issues of life and death. So go browse your local video store, or have a friend do so. You may well find your hospital has a supply. And don't forget the oldies. Many of these portray timeless themes without the high-tech graphic violence or sexual themes that beset many modern films.

Like the other art forms I've discussed in more detail, photography is something almost everyone has tried their hand at at some time. Although few of us become experts, family photographs are a never-ending source of joyful memories and connection. A powerful use for photography is the well-proven healing effect of looking at nature when confined to a bed or to the indoors, as I discussed in chapter 4. Hospitals don't always pay attention to this proven benefit, however, and the views from the wards can often be of unrelieved brick buildings, if you've got a window at all.

So it's a very good idea, if you're ill or largely confined to the indoors, to get some pictures of nature to put on your walls. See if you or a family member can find color pictures of forests or water-falls, or close-ups of trees and other growing plants. You don't have to spend a lot of money on this. You can choose a picture out of a book, and for a dollar or two have it color-copied and blown up to whatever size suits you. Then you can either frame your new artwork or simply mount it on cardboard to go on the wall.

I always try to encourage anyone who is going to have an extended stay in the hospital to bring with them their family snap-shots. Most of us have accumulated lots of pictures that are still in their packets, never seeing the light of day. A hospital bed, or even a clinic waiting room, is an ideal location for taking out all those holi-day and other snapshots and organizing them into albums. They also make a great way for getting to know your neighbors. You can now find inexpensive albums and supplementary materials to offset and highlight your pictures, and to help you create different themes and topics.

Story: One Picture Is Worth a Thousand Words

I look after a lot of young people with serious illnesses. Not only their conditions but their rigorous treatments are terribly hard on their appearance. Chemotherapy and the like causes people to lose or gain a lot of weight, shed their hair, collect more than their share of scars and other damage, quite apart from any surgical scars they often pick up along the way. Grown-ups often have it even worse; it seems their tolerance of these things is much less than children's.

I remember a patient—I'll call her Emma—who went through more than two years of such treatment. It lasted from when she was fifteen until just after her eighteenth birthday, pretty important years to a young woman on the threshold of adult life. She was also a ballet dancer, so it was especially hard on her that she had a cancer in her leg that required major surgery and prolonged lack of use.

But Emma was equal to the ordeal. Soon after I met her, she acquainted me with her family—including a rabbit and two large dogs—through photographs that she would bring with her for hospi-tal stays. Then, perhaps realizing that she was going to undergo a lot of physical changes from her treatment, she decided to document the whole process of her illness through photographs. Her photo albums soon became her personal journal, just like many of us have made of our newborn babies as they grow through infancy.

Whenever she was in the hospital, it was both moving and rewarding to share in her journey through her pictures. Although some of them were family shots, most of them were of herself, usually taken by her mother or elder sister. Some of them were pretty graphic, including pictures of her recently operated-on leg and plenty of her bald head. She had instinctively hit on the idea that seeing herself in pictures at all stages of her treatment and recovery would help her somehow put the experience *outside of herself* and so help her deal with it better.

This is a crucial aspect of the healing effect of art-making, and I can think of no better way to achieve it. I even suggested she try an idea that was first used, as far as I know, by the photographer Katie Tartakoff. Instead of taking color photos, her mother took a series of black-and-white facial portraits over a period of months, during the time she had no hair. Then she arranged for them to be blown up almost to life size, and Emma painted her scalp with all colors of the rainbow. What a wonderful example of turning physical affliction into art.

Exercise: Family Album

I invite you now to use some time—which might be hanging heavy if you're in the hospital—to create an album of family snapshots. Perhaps you're a person who has always been super-efficient at mounting all your photos; if so, you're pretty unusual. But you can still do this exercise, which is especially good fun to do with other family members. You or one of your family will need to buy a photo album, or dig one up at home, and then gather together all the pictures you can find stored in odd places, as well as any albums you've already filled up.

The idea is to collect together for mounting a body of pictures that tells a story. It may be a strictly chronological tale of your life over the past few years, or it may stretch back to childhood. It may have a theme to it, like the overcoming of illness or disability, or the story of a marriage. Like all the art-making in this book, it's important not to be concerned with the expertise of the photography, but rather to focus on the memories, and perhaps the emotional responses the pictures evoke in you. Of course the most vital thing is to share the process together.

You might decide to make collages, particularly if you have a lot of similar pictures you don't know what to do with. Try juxtaposing different images on each other and see the effect. Remember, art-making is never about going in a straight line, so don't try to stay too strictly chronological or tie yourself to a particular theme. Let your imagination roam about a good bit, and find out how quite simple everyday snaps can be transformed into beautiful collages.

Leave enough room for writing a few lines about the work on each page. More than one person may well want to do this, just like people often write collectively on a greeting card to someone having a birthday or recovering from illness. I very much hope that by now you've tried your hand at journaling; this picture-play is a marvelous and user-friendly way to create a journal of words and photos combined, about your memories, your feelings, your hopes, and even your fears. Write messages to the people in the pictures, like writing letters to them. Just keep the conversation going.

This is another quite lengthy project, and you certainly don't have to complete it at one sitting. Find a place to store it and something to hold the spare photographs. So what if they get all jumbled up—that's all the better for recreating the stories they hold.

Puppetry

Most of us at some time in our childhood made and played with puppets. Puppets are precious inanimate objects made to come alive as people and other species. They're not only works of art, they're tools for expressing thoughts and feelings. They're especially useful for communicating through a kind of third party, when you have thoughts and feelings that are hard to express.

As far as health and health care are concerned, puppets have been used a lot with children who've had serious illnesses and traumas, to allow them to express themselves more freely. Puppetry is rather like drama therapy, as discussed in chapter 7. It's a form of dramatic communication. But puppets are also just fun to make. You can build a whole family, perhaps creating one to represent each of your absent family members or friends. Or you can use them as a means of self-expression, to express all aspects of your personality and moods. And you can talk to them as friends in the wee small hours.

There are several kinds of puppets, ranging from simple stick or rod puppets to finger and hand ones, to the most sophisticated kind, string puppets or marionettes. Marionettes have an ancient and noble history; they were originally carved in the image of the Virgin Mary. I've got a considerable collection of hand and finger puppets, and I like to carry a few with me when I go on ward rounds—and not just to entertain little children! You can buy these kinds of puppets very inexpensively, but I urge you to make your own.

Exercise: Puppet-Making

To make a rod or stick family of puppets, you'll need a few simple supplies. Most of these supplies are the sort we're all trying to recycle rather than simply throw in the garbage, and I can't think of a better way to recycle used materials.

First, get yourself some brown paper bags (varying from small lunch bags to larger grocery bags). Then you'll need some kind of stick or pole. I've used at various times bamboo poles, sturdy sticks from the yard, curtain rods, and even broom handles. Once more, remember that you don't have to get hung up on exactness, in dimensions or anything else. But you'll need some kind of strut to keep your puppet erect. You'll also need some newspaper, glue, masking tape, scissors, white and colored tissue paper, and crayons. Lastly, collect and cut up some pieces of cloth from cast-off clothing, preferably in different colors. You may need to get someone to help you collect these things together, but they should all be pretty readily available.

The first thing to do is to choose two sturdy struts or rods to strap together with tape in the form of a cross, the longer one vertical and the other crossways to form the shoulder girdle and support your puppet's clothes. Now you're going to make the head and face, which is where most of your puppet's animation will come from. Use one of your lunch-size sacks for this. Crumple it up to give you the first shot at the face—the more crumpled the better to define a skin-like texture. If you cut off the bottom couple of inches, you can make your puppet's face more rounded. You may want to turn the bag inside out first if there's a lot of printing on it.

Now crumple up one sheet of newspaper at a time and use them to stuff into your puppet's head and face, shaping the features as you go. Then mount the head on the vertical pole. It's important that the pole go right up through the head's insides to make it stable. Tape the puppet's neck around the bottom, above the crossbar. You can make the facial features very three-dimensional. Use wads of colored tissue paper for the eyes, nose, ears, mouth. Don't be too literal in your choice of color—the eyes don't have to be blue and all the other features don't have to be pink. Allow yourself a little artistic license! Glue these various features in place.

Crumple up more newspaper for the hair and eyebrows, and—if you want to add them—moustache and beard. You can either crayon these the color of your choice or substitute strands of tissue paper. Now take a larger grocery bag for the puppet's body. Use more tape to strap the head and neck onto it. Pick out a large piece of cloth to wrap around it, and find a colored cotton belt for its middle. Fasten this too with tape at the back. You may want to add buttons and pockets in the form of colored paper.

You've now got the elements of your first puppet together. You need two more lunch bags for the hands. Tear their open ends into ten strips, going about halfway down the bags. Twist two together to form each finger. Cut the bottom out of each bag and stuff them lightly with wads of newspaper to form the hands. Now tape each one to the side of the body, quite high up near the shoulders.

Now sit back and admire your handiwork. Any last-minute touches you want to add? Now you get to decide who this puppet represents: a family member or friend, or maybe some facet of yourself. It only remains for you to give him or her a name, before you start on another member of your puppet family. If you find yourself creating several puppets to represent different aspects of yourself, don't hesitate to make some masculine and some feminine. After all, you want to see both the masculine and the feminine aspects of your psyche represented, don't you?

Healthy Habits

I want to talk to you a bit about staying motivated as an artist. It comes down to making it a habit, or ritual, like brushing your teeth in the morning. Once you establish the habit, and your art in its many facets and ways of self-expression becomes your friend, then it will be much easier to stick with it, because you'll make it a priority. You'll come to feel deprived of the chance to make art if you put it aside for any length of time. You'll miss it like a good friend. After all, good habits are as hard to break as bad ones.

Exercise: Taking Inventory

This is a two-part exercise to help you keep your motivation. The first thing to do—and you started on it earlier in this chapter—is to take inventory. Collect together all the works of art you've created over the course of this book, and make a list of all the things you've accomplished, plus the projects you are still working on. I've given you the format for doing this below. Use your workbook for this, leaving a few lines under each heading. I also suggest some questions you may want to ask yourself about your art-making activities, and the effects they've had on you.

Projects I have tried _____

Projects I have yet to complete _____

Other projects I want to try _____

Projects that involve several people _____

Titles for my works of art _____

My favorite activities _____

My least favorite _____

Why? What gets in my way? _____

(Example) is helpful because _____

The hard part is _____

The fulfilling part is _____

What have I learned from all this? _____

How has my overall health been affected? _____

Exercise: Weekly Schedule

The other half of this exercise is to set up for yourself a schedule of art activities. The easiest thing is to use your workbook to draw up a plan for the next four weeks. You may want to have one session each day, or even two. You'll also need to decide how much time you're going to spend, and try to stick to it. Think about this a bit, so you don't get overambitious and find you're letting yourself down. It may be a good idea to gradually increase the time you spend, depending on your circumstances.

Here's an example of how to lay things out:

Monday A.M.	(Date)	(Activity)	(Comments)
Monday P.M.	(Date)	(Activity)	(Comments)
Tuesday A.M.	(Date)	(Activity)	(Comments)
Tuesday P.M.	(Date)	(Activity)	(Comments)

And so on: It's a good plan to vary your activities, interweaving projects that are easy to accomplish with more challenging ones. Use the space under "Comments" to add a note about the time spent, and any reactions—memories and images, thoughts and feelings—that come up during the time you pursue these different activities. Note any changes you experience in your health—in your body, mind, and spirit, and in your relationships—over time.

Times of Celebration

In addition to drawing up a weekly or monthly schedule, there will be particular days or occasions you want to recognize by means of a special celebration. We all have times during the year for these. Some are common to many of us, like Thanksgiving, Hanukkah, or Christmas. Others, like birthdays, are specific to families. Then there are those one-shot occasions that happen as a part of our life's circumstances. In the day-to-day world, these may be related to the particular success of a child at school, or to obtaining a new job you were going after, or to moving into a new house. In relation to illness, there are also special days that should be marked, such as the end of a long and arduous course of treatment, or recovery from surgery, or getting discharged from the hospital after a long stay as an inpatient. And of course you don't have to have a special reason to celebrate. Random acts of rejoicing are as glorious as random acts of kindness.

These times are ideal for celebrating with some form of art-making activity that will serve to mark the occasion, as well as to display your newly acquired skills. Such significant occasions deserve to be observed with the kind of symbolic recognition that art lends itself to. On these occasions, nothing beats a piece of your very own artwork as a gift to a loved one, or indeed to yourself if you've just overcome some particular life challenge.

So I suggest you spend a few minutes reflecting on and making a list in a prominent spot in your workbook of such times in your own life—those that you will want to mark on a regular basis, and those that happen only once. Then take the time to give some thought to how you want to symbolize these moments of passage in your life.

Last Thoughts

As a closing act of contemplation, I invite you to take a look at your whole life to date, as well as your expectations for the future. If illness or disability has slowed you or a loved one down a bit—or a lot—in recent times, you may well have found yourself reflecting on the larger issues of your life that have hitherto been sidelined in your busy day-to-day life. Serious illness can serve to remind you of the really important issues of life and can put a fresh perspective on things. You may have found yourself contemplating such thoughts as the true purpose of life, and how we as a society could make this a more rational, safe, and loving world. You may want to commit yourself to making some changes in the way you live your own life, what your priorities are, and how you distribute the precious gift of your time.

Exercise: Priorities

So here's your chance to put these thoughts and ideas on paper. Put these open-ended questions in your workbook, to reflect on and write about as the mood takes you. Each one deserves at least a couple of sentences, and there may well be other similar ones you want to add. I don't expect you to finish this exercise all at one sitting. It's better to come back to it from time to time, filling in the gaps and dwelling on the issues that come up for you. Don't forget to add a note each time of the date, location, and your circumstances.

1. In one or two sentences, what is the true purpose of my life?

2. What are my core beliefs and principles?

3. What have I learned from my acquaintance with illness or disability?

4. What have I learned from bringing art and art-making back into my life?

5. How do I want people to think of me when I'm gone?

6. What would I like to leave behind to be remembered by?

7. When I envision a more rational world, what does it look like?

8. How can I contribute to making this world a better place?

9. What help do I need, and how can I get it?

10. What are my six top priorities for the next six months?

I hope you've enjoyed reading this book and practicing the many exercises. I sincerely trust that from now on you will always:

1. Count your blessings, especially on days when you don't feel like you have any.

2. Withhold judgment of people, particularly yourself.

3. Acknowledge that there's a purpose to all illness and affliction, even though it may often seem hard to fathom.

4. Recognize that every one of us is an artist, a creator.

5. Practice your new art-making skills every day—for your greater health and well-being!

References

Achterberg , J. 1992. *Woman as Healer*. Boston: Shambhala.

Achterberg, J., and G. F. Lawlis. 1984. *Imagery and Disease*. Champaign, Ill.: Institute for Personality and Ability Testing.

Adams, P., and M. Mylander. 1998. *Gesundheit!* Rochester, Vt.: Healing Arts Press.

Ader, R. 1981. *Psychoneuroimmunology*. New York: Academic Press.

Baldwin, C. 1991. *Life's Companion: Journal Writing as a Spiritual Quest*. New York: Bantam Books.

Berk, L. S., S. A. Tan, W. F. Fry, et al. 1989. Neuroendocrine and stress hormone changes during mirthful laughter. *American Journal of Medical Science* 298:390–396.

Bertman, S. L., ed. 1999. *Grief and the Healing Arts: Creativity as Therapy*. Amityville, N.Y.: Baywood Publishing Company.

Block, J., J. Swanson, J. R. Mott, and C. Wallace. 1992. *The Healing "I."* Gainesville, Fla.: The Write Solutions.

Brody, H. 1987. *Stories of Sickness*. New Haven, Conn.: Yale University Press.

Cameron, J. 1992. *The Artist's Way: A Spiritual Path to Higher Creativity*. New York: Tarcher/Putnam.

Campbell, D. 1997. *The Mozart Effect*. New York: Avon Books.

Coles, R. 1993. "A Special Interview with Robert Coles: How to Look at a Mountain." *Art News*, 91–99.

Cousins N. 1979. *Anatomy of an Illness*. New York: Bantam/Norton.

Cousins, N. 1989. *Head First: The Biology of Hope*. New York: Dutton.

Csikszentmihalyi, M. 1990. *Flow: The Psychology of Optimal Experience*. New York: Harper & Row.

Dienstfrey, H. 1991. *Where the Mind Meets the Body*. New York: Harper.

Ellison, G. 1996. *House Renovation as a Recurrent Motif in Dreams*. Unpublished doctoral dissertation.

Emunah, R. 1994. *Acting for Real: Drama Therapy Process, Technique, and Performance*. Levittown, Pa.: Brunner/Mazel.

Erikson, E. 1950. *Childhood and Society*. New York: Norton.

Foster, S. L., ed. 1995. *Choreographing History*. Bloomington, Ind.: Indiana University Press.

Fox, J. 1995. *Finding What You Didn't Lose: Expressing Your Truth and Creativity Through Poem-Making*. New York: Tarcher/Putnam.

Fox, J. 1997. *Poetic Medicine: The Healing Art of Poem-Making*. New York: Tarcher/Putnam.

Fromm, E. 1957. *The Art of Loving*. London: Mandala.

Fry, W. F. 1977. The respiratory components of mirthful laughter. *Journal of Biological Psychology* 19:39–50

Fry, W. F., and W. A. Salameh, eds. 1993. *Advances in Humor and Psychology*. Sarasota, Fla.: Professional Resources Press.

Garfield, L. M. 1987. *Sound Medicine: Healing with Music, Voice and Song*. Berkeley, Calif.: Celestial Arts.

Goffman, E. 1961. *Encounters: Two Studies in the Sociology of Interaction*. Indianapolis, Ind.: Bobbs-Merrill.

Goldberg, N. 1986. *Writing Down the Bones*. Boston: Shambhala.

Goldstein, J. H., and P. McGhee, eds. 1983. *Handbook of Humor Research*. New York: Springer-Verlag.

Graham-Pole, J. 1996. Children, death, and poetry. *Journal of Poetry Therapy* 9:129–141.

Homan, S. 1994. The theatre in medicine. *International Journal of Arts Medicine* 3:26–29.

Horace. 23 B.C. *Odes* Book I, Ode I.

Hospital Audiences, Inc. 220 W. 42nd Street, New York, N.Y. 10036. (212) 575–7676.

Ivker, R., and E. Zorensky. 1997. *Thriving.* New York: Random House.

Johnstone, K. 1992. *Impro: Improvisation and the Theatre.* New York: Routledge.

Kabat-Zinn, J. 1994. *Wherever You Go, There You Are.* New York: Hyperion.

Kaminski, J., and W. Hall. 1996. The effect of soothing music on neonatal behavioral states in the hospital newborn nursery. *Neonatal Network* 15:45–52.

Kaptchuk, T. J. 1983. *The Web That Has No Weaver: Understanding Chinese Medicine.* New York: Congdon & Weed.

Lefcourt, H. M., K. Davidson-Katz, et al. 1990. Humor and immune-system functioning. *International Journal of Humor Research* 3: 305–322.

Levine, S. 1997. *A Year to Live: How to Live This Year as if It Were Your Last.* New York: Bell Tower.

Lewis, C. S. 1960. *The Four Loves.* Orlando, Fla.: Harcourt, Brace & Company.

Lingerman, H. A. 1995. *The Healing Energies of Music.* Wheaton, Ill.: Quest Books.

Malchiodi, C. A. 1999. *Medical Art Therapy with Adults.* London and Philadelphia: Jessica Kingsley.

McNiff, S. 1992. *Art as Medicine: Creating a Therapy of the Imagination.* Boston: Shambhala.

Milne, A. A. 1926. *Winnie-the-Pooh.* London: E. P. Dutton.

Miró, J. 1938. *Je reve d'un grand atelier.* Paris: XX Siecle.

Nachmanovitch, S. 1990. *Free Play: Improvisation in Life and Art.* New York: Tarcher/Putnam.

Nightingale, F. 1859. *Notes on Nursing: What It Is and What It Is Not.* London: Harrison and Sons.

Ornish, D. 1998. *Love and Survival: 8 Pathways to Intimacy and Health.* New York: Harper Perennial.

Pennebaker, J. 1997. *Opening Up: The Healing Power of Confiding in Others.* New York: Avon Books.

Pennebaker, J. 1997. *Opening Up: The Healing Power of Expressing Emotions*. New York: Guilford Press.

Pert, C. 1997. *Molecules of Emotion*. New York: Scribner.

Robinson, V. M. 1991. *Humor and the Health Professions: The Therapeutic Use of Humor in Health Care*. Thorofare, N.J.: Slack

SARK. 1991. *A Creative Companion: How to Free the Creative Spirit*. Berkeley, Calif.: Celestial Arts.

Samuels, M., and M. Rockwood Lane. 1998. *Creative Healing*. San Francisco: HarperSanFrancisco.

Schroeder-Sheker, T. 1994. Music for the dying: a personal account of the new field of music thanatology—history, theories, and clinical narratives. *Journal of Holistic Nursing* 12:83–99.

Siegel, B. 1986. *Love, Medicine, and Miracles*. New York: Harper.

Simons, T. R. 1996. *Feng Shui Step by Step*. New York: Random House.

Simonton, C., S. Matthews-Simonton, and J. Creighton. 1981. *Getting Well Again*. New York: Bantam.

Spear, W. 1995. *Feng Shui Made Easy*. San Francisco: HarperSanFrancisco.

Spiegel, D., J. R. Bloom, H. C. Kraemer, and E. Gottheil. 1989. Effect of psychosocial treatment on survival of patients with metastatic breast cancer. *Lancet* 1:888–891.

Standley, J. 1991. *Music Techniques in Therapy, Counseling, and Special Education*. St. Louis, Mo.: MMB Music.

Toombs, S. K. 1993. *The Meaning of Illness*. Norwell, Mass.: Kluwer Academic Publishers.

Ulrich, R. S. 1984. View through a window may influence recovery from surgery. *Science* 224:420–421.

Warren, B., ed. 1997. *Using the Creative Arts in Therapy: A Practical Introduction*. 2nd edition. New York: Routledge.

More New Harbinger Titles

MULTIPLE CHEMICAL SENSITIVITY

Provides step-by-step advice for coping with MCS, including taking steps to make your home safe, getting professional help, and mobilizing the support of family and friends.   *Item MCS $16.95*

A SURVIVOR'S GUIDE TO BREAST CANCER

A clinical psychologist who treats people with life-threatening illnesses details her own struggle with breast cancer, from the initial discovery of a lump through treatment and back to full health.   *Item BRST $13.95*

I'LL TAKE CARE OF YOU

Helps family caregivers cope with uncomfortable thoughts and feelings, avoid burnout, set boundaries, and find ways of meeting their own needs. *Item CARE $12.95*

LIVING WELL WITH A HIDDEN DISABILITY

Provides a wealth of resources for healthy living, including advice on navigating the health care system and suggestions for strengthening the body, mind, and soul.   *Item HID $15.95*

WINNING AGAINST RELAPSE

A structured program teaches you how to monitor symptoms and respond to them in a way that reduces or eliminates the possibility of relapse. *Item WIN $14.95*

THE CHRONIC PAIN CONTROL WORKBOOK

A team of specialists in all areas of pain management detail the treatment strategies for managing and recovering from chronic pain. *Item PN2 $18.95*

Call **toll-free 1-800-748-6273** to order. Have your Visa or Mastercard number ready. Or send a check for the titles you want to New Harbinger Publications, 5674 Shattuck Avenue, Oakland, CA 94609. Include $3.80 for the first book and 75¢ for each additional book to cover shipping and handling. (California residents please include appropriate sales tax.) Allow four to six weeks for delivery.

Prices subject to change without notice.

Some Other New Harbinger Self-Help Titles

Multiple Chemical Sensitivity: A Survival Guide, $16.95
Dancing Naked, $14.95
Why Are We Still Fighting, $15.95
From Sabotage to Success, $14.95
Parkinson's Disease and the Art of Moving, $15.95
A Survivor's Guide to Breast Cancer, $13.95
Men, Women, and Prostate Cancer, $15.95
Make Every Session Count: Getting the Most Out of Your Brief Therapy, $10.95
Virtual Addiction, $12.95
After the Breakup, $13.95
Why Can't I Be the Parent I Want to Be?, $12.95
The Secret Message of Shame, $13.95
The OCD Workbook, $18.95
Tapping Your Inner Strength, $13.95
Binge No More, $14.95
When to Forgive, $12.95
Practical Dreaming, $12.95
Healthy Baby, Toxic World, $15.95
Making Hope Happen, $14.95
I'll Take Care of You, $12.95
Survivor Guilt, $14.95
Children Changed by Trauma, $13.95
Understanding Your Child's Sexual Behavior, $12.95
The Self-Esteem Companion, $10.95
The Gay and Lesbian Self-Esteem Book, $13.95
Making the Big Move, $13.95
How to Survive and Thrive in an Empty Nest, $13.95
Living Well with a Hidden Disability, $15.95
Overcoming Repetitive Motion Injuries the Rossiter Way, $15.95
What to Tell the Kids About Your Divorce, $13.95
The Divorce Book, Second Edition, $15.95
Claiming Your Creative Self: True Stories from the Everyday Lives of Women, $15.95
Six Keys to Creating the Life You Desire, $19.95
Taking Control of TMJ, $13.95
What You Need to Know About Alzheimer's, $15.95
Winning Against Relapse: A Workbook of Action Plans for Recurring Health and Emotional Problems, $14.95
Facing 30: Women Talk About Constructing a Real Life and Other Scary Rites of Passage, $12.95
The Worry Control Workbook, $15.95
Wanting What You Have: A Self-Discovery Workbook, $18.95
When Perfect Isn't Good Enough: Strategies for Coping with Perfectionism, $13.95
Earning Your Own Respect: A Handbook of Personal Responsibility, $12.95
High on Stress: A Woman's Guide to Optimizing the Stress in Her Life, $13.95
Infidelity: A Survival Guide, $13.95
Stop Walking on Eggshells, $14.95
Consumer's Guide to Psychiatric Drugs, $16.95
The Fibromyalgia Advocate: Getting the Support You Need to Cope with Fibromyalgia and Myofascial Pain, $18.95
Healing Fear: New Approaches to Overcoming Anxiety, $16.95
Working Anger: Preventing and Resolving Conflict on the Job, $12.95
Sex Smart: How Your Childhood Shaped Your Sexual Life and What to Do About It, $14.95
You Can Free Yourself From Alcohol & Drugs, $13.95
Amongst Ourselves: A Self-Help Guide to Living with Dissociative Identity Disorder, $14.95
Healthy Living with Diabetes, $13.95
Dr. Carl Robinson's Basic Baby Care, $10.95
Better Boundaries: Owning and Treasuring Your Life, $13.95
Goodbye Good Girl, $12.95
Fibromyalgia & Chronic Myofascial Pain Syndrome, $19.95
The Depression Workbook: Living With Depression and Manic Depression, $17.95
Self-Esteem, Second Edition, $13.95
Angry All the Time: An Emergency Guide to Anger Control, $12.95
When Anger Hurts, $13.95
Perimenopause, $16.95
The Relaxation & Stress Reduction Workbook, Fourth Edition, $17.95
The Anxiety & Phobia Workbook, Second Edition, $18.95
I Can't Get Over It, A Handbook for Trauma Survivors, Second Edition, $16.95
Messages: The Communication Skills Workbook, Second Edition, $15.95
Thoughts & Feelings, Second Edition, $18.95
Depression: How It Happens, How It's Healed, $14.95
The Deadly Diet, Second Edition, $14.95
The Power of Two, $15.95

Call **toll free, 1-800-748-6273**, or log on to our online bookstore at **www.newharbinger.com** to order. Have your Vis
or Mastercard number ready. Or send a check for the titles you want to New Harbinger Publications, Inc., 5674 Sha
tuck Ave., Oakland, CA 94609. Include $3.80 for the first book and 75¢ for each additional book, to cover shipping an
handling. (California residents please include appropriate sales tax.) Allow two to five weeks for delivery.

Prices subject to change without notice.